SECRETS OF HEALING THE BRAIN

NATURAL OPTIONS IN NEUROLOGY,
PSYCHIATRY, AND TRAUMA

Secrets of
Healing
the Brain

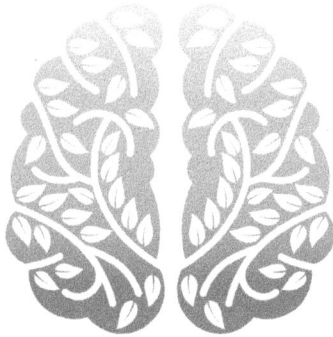

SHADY J. SROUR

Foreword by Hanna A. Srour, MD

To Jude and Leo, I love You with all my heart.

CONTENTS

—1—

Herbal Medicine and Neurological Health

1

—2—

Important Issues

57

—3—

Conditions

105

—4—

Public Policies

143

FOREWORD

As a board-certified family physician for more than 20 years, my view that conventional medicine was the end-all and be-all of medicine has changed. Today, I consider conventional medicine to be a part of a vast medical knowledge that humans possess. I see that the culture of conventional medicine contains elements of competition and a view of its superiority over other traditional medical systems. Conventional medicine needs more humility, and should be part of the picture, but not the entire picture of medical knowledge. We need to be more humble in this time of history and respect and honor the historical human medical knowledge that was built upon thousands of years of tradition.

I have known Shady for many years. I see him as a deep, committed medical investigator. He searches not only the medical literature, but also uses his life and his body as a laboratory for expanding knowledge related to healing. He is a truth seeker. Shady is a Palestinian, born in Italy, raised and educated in the United States, and later on lived in Israel/Palestine, giving him a multi-cultural experience.

He is a human being who looked with deep curiosity into his own suffering from medical disability. He used that challenge and understood that pain and suffering is a path that our body uses to guide itself toward healing. Our responsibility is not to simply suppress symptoms, but more importantly to create the conditions that support fundamental healing.

In this book, Shady shares his valuable experience and knowledge of more than 20 years. Medical clinicians who are looking for potential methods to support our patients will find this book valuable. Patients who read this work may find comfort and facilitate their healing.

Hanna A. Srour, MD
Family Medicine Physician

ACKNOWLEDGMENTS

I want to thank my brothers, Habib and Andre. I love you both so much. To my parents, thanks for bringing me into this world. And thank you so much for all of the support over the years. I want to thank my children, Leo and Jude, for inspiring me every day. It is an absolute honor to be your father. I want to thank my Uncle Rabia. I appreciate you so much. And a huge thanks to my cousin and my friend, Hanna, for such a long and enduring friendship. That friendship helped me throughout challenging times over the years. I also want to thank Dina. You have been such a meaningful friend to me, and I appreciate you. Nader, my friend, thank you for the countless hours of conversations and deep dialogue. Your kindness and generosity always move me deeply. Thanks are not enough.

To all of my friends from my days at Southwest College of Naturopathic Medicine, I still think of you often. We will always be family.

To Susan Bruck, my editor, you have been wonderful to work with. You've helped transform the manuscript and have helped present my ideas in a more polished and beautiful way. This work wouldn't be possible without you. Thank you.

My deepest gratitude to Jasmine Hromjak, your design work was instrumental in this work's creation. Many thanks

To Chad Raisch, Bonnie Buddendeck, and Professor Jeffrey Langland, you were extraordinary examples of the art of teaching. I was honored to be taught by you.

A big thanks to Dr. Dietrich Klinghardt and Dr. Savely Yurkovsky-I learned so much from both of you.

Thank you to Monica de Sa. I don't think this work would have come to fruition without your influence in my life. And to Dr. Akhlas Ismail, thank you so much.

A deep thanks to the following people, whose work has profoundly influenced me: Dr. Peter R. Breggin, Dr. James Gordon, Dr. Bessel van der Kolk, Dr. James M. Greenblatt, Kayla Grossmann, RN, Dr. Mark Millar, Dr. Ramani Durvasula, Dr. Elaine N. Aron, Dr. Gabor Maté, Dr. Joe Dispenza, Pete Walker, Sarah Peyton, Anita Moorjani, Dr. Zach Bush, Robert F. Kennedy Jr., Dr. Joseph Mercola, Dr. Baxter D. Montgomery, Dr. Joel Fuhrman, Dr. Alan Goldhamer, Dr. Caldwell B. Esselstyn Jr., Dr. Dean Ornish, Dr. John A. McDougall, Dr. Neal D. Barnard, Dr. Michael Greger, Ralph Nader, Wim Hof, Dr. Devra Lee Davis, Dr. Milton Mills, Dr. Michael T. Murray, and Dr. Joseph Pizzorno. There are more, and I thank them also.

Thanks to Ingram Spark and to Reedsy for their critical roles in bringing this book to life. And gratitude toward Amo-Te Fotografia in Ponte de Lima, Portugal for their kindness and talent.

Finally, gratitude toward God for getting me here and for this most interesting journey of life.

INTRODUCTION

Modern conventional neurology and psychiatry require new methods of addressing the conditions practitioners deal with regularly. Techniques should have strong efficacy and safety and attempt to address the underlying causes of the conditions rather than just the symptoms. The purpose of this work is to demonstrate, with a high level of evidence, that Natural Medicine can play a fundamental role in the prevention and treatment of neuropsychiatric conditions. Neurology, in the context of this work, encompasses a broad definition, which includes not only traditional neurology but also psychiatry, since the neurological system is involved in both fields of medicine. In Chapter 1, Herbal Medicine, with an emphasis on neurological applications, is discussed. In Chapter 2, I review many vital issues that impact neuropsychiatric health. Chapter 3 presents a short reference guide for protocols for addressing various specific conditions. And finally, Chapter 4 delves into public policy and its impact on the brain. The work is really meant to be taken as a whole, and the information provided is much more valuable when used in that way. That being said, feel free to jump to the sections which are of particular interest. But I strongly recommend you review the entire work for maximum benefits.

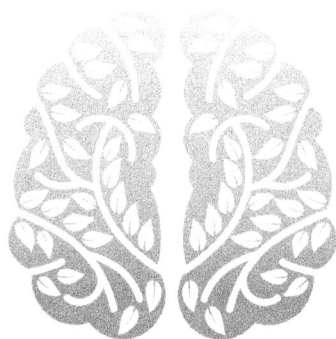

CHAPTER 1

Herbal Medicine and Neurological Health

Allium sativum (GARLIC)

Garlic has broad applications in herbal medicine. These include numerous multi-system effects, including anti-cancer, anti-atherosclerotic, immune-boosting, anti-allergy, anti-parasitic, anti-epileptic, antiviral, anti-fungal, and antibacterial properties.[1] Garlic has an important place in the treatment and prevention of neurological disorders. In that regard, there is a clear connection between vascular disease and neurological disease since healthy brain function depends on healthy vascular function. In addition, through reduction in inflammation, garlic may be beneficial with respect to multiple sclerosis, Alzheimer's disease, and Parkinson's disease.[2] Garlic appears to improve flow-mediated dilation and, therefore, may be useful in ischemic stroke patients.[3] In general, it has a beneficial effect on the vascular system, including a reduction in stroke risk, reduction in blood pressure, and improved lipid and glucose levels[4] Finally, there is additional evidence suggesting that garlic may be beneficial with respect to Alzheimer's disease.[5]

With such a broad range of potential beneficial effects, as well as garlic's relative safety and wide availability, it is logical to incorporate garlic into the diet as a component of neurological disease prevention and treatment. In cases where infections may be involved in neurological disorders, garlic may provide support against various infectious agents.

Based on historical experience in nutrition, it may be a mistake to focus on isolating one or more compounds from garlic in an attempt to create more refined products. The safety of the refined products may be reduced compared to whole garlic, and efficacy may also be adversely affected. One need not look beyond the historical experience with synthetic isolated beta carotene versus whole carrots to understand the issues involved here. As part of a complete and individualized program dealing with neurological issues, incorporating organic whole garlic into the diet seems wiser than using standardized extracts or isolated garlic compounds. Incorporating up to 3 cloves of raw garlic per day appears advisable for optimal neurological health.[6-7] For refined garlic products, follow the manufacturer's instructions. One should attempt to eat garlic in the middle of a meal to avoid irritating the digestive tract. If digestive upset occurs, the dosage should be reduced or the garlic discontinued completely.

Garlic may interact with blood-thinning medications, and care must be taken to avoid significant side effects.[8] There are numerous other potential drug interactions.[9] Avoid use prior to surgery. Use garlic cautiously in people with bleeding disorders. Only utilize it in normal food quantities in children, pregnant women, and while breast-feeding. Body odor and garlic breath, along with various digestive symptoms, are some possible side effects. In general, garlic's safety profile is good.

Bacopa monnieri (BACOPA)

Bacopa is a plant used in traditional Ayurvedic Medicine. It can improve cognitive function and provide neuroprotective effects.[1-2] Considering the effects of Bacopa on neuro-inflammation, the potential therapeutic possibilities are broad. Bacopa's anti-inflammatory effect within the nervous system opens the door to its potential use in the treatment of Alzheimer's disease, schizophrenia, multiple sclerosis, depression, Parkinson's disease, bipolar disorder, and anxiety.[3] This herb also has tremendous potential as a useful therapeutic agent in children and teenagers with respect to improving behavior, cognitive abilities, and attention deficit.[4] This herb should certainly be considered an excellent option for various neurological conditions. Follow the manufacturer's instructions on dosage and safety considerations for whatever preparation you use.[5-6] One may use 1 cup of the tea up to 3 times per day (pour 1 liter of boiling water on 15 grams of the herb and steep for 15 minutes). The herb should not be utilized in people with hyperthyroidism. There are also significant drug interactions. In general, the safety profile is good. Fatigue, stomach cramps, dry mouth, nausea, and change in bowel movements are some possible side effects.

Brassica oleracea (CABBAGE, KALE, CAULIFLOWER, BROCCOLI, COLLARD GREENS, BRUSSELS SPROUTS, KOHLRABI)

This is a species which includes a variety of edible plants, such as cabbage, kale, cauliflower, broccoli, collard greens, Brussels sprouts, and kohlrabi. These foods are profoundly beneficial components of a healthy diet. In terms of neurological applications, the juice from broccoli sprouts may have potential utility in the prevention and/or treatment of Alzheimer's disease.[1] This evidence is quite preliminary (from a cell-based model), but with minimal risk as part of a healthy whole-food plant-based diet, it would seem logical to incorporate these foods for promoting general health, including neurological health.

A significant focus has been on sulforaphane, a substance indirectly formed from the consumption of these vegetables. Glucoraphanin, in the presence of myrosinase, is converted to sulforaphane. Consumption of these vegetables raw will maximize sulforaphane formation. Sulforaphane is potentially useful in the prevention and/or treatment of Parkinson's disease, Alzheimer's disease, autism, traumatic brain injury, and stroke; this substance appears to be neuroprotective and anti-inflammatory.[2] In autism, the positive effect of sulforaphane may be profound.[3-5] Its safety profile is excellent.[6] Close blood sugar monitoring is necessary for diabetics, as blood sugar may be lowered by *Brassica oleracea.* Those with hypothyroidism should be cautious and ensure adequate iodine intake along with cruciferous vegetable intake. There are many possible drug interactions. In summary, the wide variety of vegetables from this species should be strongly considered for use in herbal medicine with respect to neurological conditions.

Camelia sinensis (BLACK TEA, WHITE TEA, GREEN TEA, PU'ER TEA, OOLONG TEA)

This species refers to several different types of tea which come from the same plant but undergo different forms of processing. Black tea, white tea, green tea, Pu'er tea, and oolong tea are examples of teas derived from *Camelia sinensis*. This species appears to have significant and broad potential use in neurology. Green tea has potential benefits in the prevention and treatment of cognitive dysfunction.[1] Tea may help prevent stroke, in addition to providing neuroprotection and reduction in inflammation.[2] There appears to be a broadly beneficial effect on general health from tea consumption. *Camelia sinensis* may provide benefits with respect to the prevention of Parkinson's disease.[3] It may also be beneficial after a Parkinson's disease diagnosis as a viable treatment option.[4] With respect to Alzheimer's disease, *Camelia sinensis* has potential for both preventative and therapeutic uses.[5] In multiple sclerosis, there is also evidence supporting the potential therapeutic use of *Camelia sinensis*.[6] With respect to amyotrophic lateral sclerosis (ALS), Pu'er tea has exciting potential for both preventative and therapeutic benefits.[7] Safety and dosage information should be considered.[8-10] It's safety profile is good. Caffeine content should be considered, because caffeine consumption may lead to side effects including anxiety, digestive issues, insomnia, and heart palpitations. Avoid use with eating disorders, ulcers, hypertension, pregnancy, diabetes, and anxiety. Also avoid use before surgeries. There are numerous drug interactions. For green or black tea, one can drink 1-2 cups daily. Dosages for green tea are sometimes much higher. However, the likelihood of side effects from caffeine will increase proportional to the dosage. For other preparations, follow manufacturer's instructions. In summary, *Camelia sinensis* has remarkable possibilities for broad use in the application of herbal medicine in neurology.

Cannabis sativa (HEMP, MARIJUANA)

Cannabidiol (CBD) is a substance which is present in *Cannabis sativa*. It can be derived from hemp or from marijuana. This author recommends avoiding chronic significant consumption of Tetrahydrocannabinol (THC) in cases of schizophrenia and dissociation. It is beyond the scope of this work to thoroughly discuss the use of higher THC-containing substances in terms of neurology and psychiatry. However, an overview of CBD use will be included here. When utilizing CBD, full-spectrum CBD products (while still containing as close to zero THC as possible) are generally preferable.

CBD Isolate (which only contains CBD) may have utility in specific circumstances. Broad-spectrum CBD products, which contain a variety of substances but have zero THC, may also have utility in specific circumstances. Again, in general, full-spectrum CBD products are recommended.

Cannabidiol may have potential benefits in epilepsy and Alzheimer's disease.[1] In addition, it has potential benefits as an anti-anxiety, neuro-protective, and anti-psychotic substance.[2] In dissociation associated with trauma, CBD has a potential application because of its anti-psychotic properties. There is also a potential for use in COVID-19. One scientific review concludes that there is potential benefit in anxiety, addiction (substance abuse), and psychosis.[3]

There is some evidence that CBD may have utility in treating PTSD.[4] Caution is advised, however, because the level of evidence is not particularly strong at the time of writing. That being the case, I do believe that CBD has a wide potential for use in neurological and psychological disorders.

Up to 1500 mg per day of CBD seems to be reasonably safe in adults.[5] However, it is very common to use far lower dosages. The safety profile is good, but irritability, nausea, and sleepiness are possible side effects. It is important to note that there may be a possible increased risk of suicidal behavior or ideation. Check with your healthcare provider and pharmacist to prevent undesirable drug/supplement interactions and to ensure safety if you have any underlying health conditions. Caution is warranted with mixing sedatives and CBD and in people with preexisting liver conditions. It is important to note that there are potential legal issues related to CBD, depending on where you live, and you should be aware of these prior to use.

Centella asiatica (GOTU KOLA, ASIATIC PENNYWORT)

This plant is commonly referred to as Gotu Kola or Asiatic Pennywort. It provides neuroprotection against the effects of betaamyloid and also exhibits activity against amyloidogenesis, and is, therefore, potentially useful for both the prevention and treatment of Alzheimer's disease.[1-2] With Parkinson's disease, there is exciting in vitro evidence of the preventative effect of *Centella asiatica*.[3] This research demonstrated the herb's ability to prevent the alpha-synuclein aggregation that is typical in the disease. In poststroke cognitive dysfunction, this herb could offer potential benefits.[4] Finally, the plant has tremendous potential for use as both a neuroprotective agent and also in cases where neuroregeneration would be beneficial.[5-6] This makes it theoretically useful in many situations in neurology which call for an herb with such properties. In conclusion, this herb should be seriously considered by healthcare practitioners for use in numerous neurological conditions.

Dosage and safety information should be considered.[7-12] Follow the manufacturer's instructions for dosage related to specific preparations. For the powdered herb, adults may use up to 1000 mg three times per day (in vegan capsules). Overall, its safety profile is excellent. Stomach pain and nausea are possible side effects. Rarely, liver damage may occur. Avoid use in pregnancy and lactation. Dizziness can be a side effect of an overdose. Caution should be exercised in using it with anticoagulant medications. Photosensitivity is possible with use. Children under 2 years of age should not take gotu kola. Avoid use prior to surgery. There are numerous drug interactions.

Chamaemelum nobile (ENGLISH/ROMAN CHAMOMILE) or *Matricaria chamomilla* (GERMAN CHAMOMILE)

There are two species commonly referred to as "chamomile." The taxonomy on this issue is complicated, however, to keep it simple, it is sufficient to state that these related herbs (although different species) come from the same family and can both be referred to as "chamomile." This herb has a wide variety of uses in herbal medicine, including treatment of fever, digestive problems (gastritis, nausea, vomiting), wound healing (topical), gingivitis (mouthwash), inflammatory conditions, insomnia, pain, epilepsy, muscle spasms, agitation, infection, and sore throat.[1-5] Chamomile should be strongly considered as a treatment option for Generalized Anxiety Disorder (GAD).[6-8]

Chamomile has neuroprotective effects and may be beneficial in treating autism.[9] It must be noted, however, that with respect to autism, the research used an isolated compound (luteolin) from chamomile and combined it with quercetin and rutin to achieve the results.

There is evidence supporting the use of topical chamomile for treating migraines.[10] The use of this herb internally in migraine headaches should be encouraged, particularly for its effect on nausea and vomiting.

Patients with epilepsy who wish to minimize or eliminate medication use may benefit from chamomile, but care needs to be taken to maximize seizure control with the goal of minimizing medications safely.[11] In conventional medicine, there is constant fear surrounding the use of herbal medicine. This fear tends to discourage the use of natural therapies in order to support the use of conventional medications. While control of epilepsy is vital, this should not discourage the careful use of herbal medicine, which can potentially provide seizure control while allowing for a reduction in medication. Avoiding long-term side effects and improving quality of life must be prioritized when searching for proper treatments, and this will put the consideration of more natural treatments into perspective. Herbal medicine, whole-food, plant-based nutrition, and lifestyle changes (exercise, sunshine, sleep) can reduce the side effects of medications by allowing reduction and sometimes elimination of medications (depending on the condition and particular situation). These natural remedies should not be ignored as a result of fear, particularly in serious and dangerous conditions such as epilepsy.

I have observed the significant effectiveness of chamomile in improving muscle spasticity, difficulty with movement, and insomnia. While certainly anecdotal, this experience has had a profound influence on my belief in this herb's potential for use in serious neurological conditions. Chamomile should be strongly considered for use in multiple sclerosis, epilepsy, and any neurological condition requiring an anti-inflammatory and calming effect. Its effect is strong yet gentle. Side effects are minimal, with the exception of a possible allergy to chamomile itself. Numerous drug interactions are possible and use should be stopped prior to surgery.[12] Follow the manufacturer's instructions for the dosage of various preparations. For infusions, 1 cup boiling water can be poured on 1 teaspoon of dried herb (allow 10 minutes steep time). Up to 3 cups per day can be drunk of this infusion. This is a very safe herb to utilize in neurological practice and should command the deepest respect of those working with neurological conditions.

Cinnamomum verum and *Cinnamomum cassia* (CINNAMON)

Cinnamon refers generally to either *Cinnamomum verum* or *Cinnamomum cassia*. Cinnamaldehyde is present in both species, however, only *Cinnamomum cassia* contains coumarin (associated with liver toxicity).[1] The review article referenced here discusses the various mechanisms through which *Cinnamomum verum* appears to have strong potential for treating multiple sclerosis. Unfortunately, this theory is based on animal research, which is not ethical. There is a need for human clinical research using *Cinnamomum verum* for multiple sclerosis, and there should be an immediate end to animal research/testing. While the review discusses cinnamon's effect on protecting the blood-brain barrier, modulating neuroinflammation, and regulating the immune system with respect to mechanisms of action in multiple sclerosis, this information does not justify the ethically problematic research used to gather such information.

With respect to general neurological health and wellness, cinnamon is neuro-protective and has anti-neuroinflammatory activity.[2] The anti-neuroinflammatory effect should occur with both *Cinnamomum verum* and *Cinnamomum cassia*, since cinnamaldehyde was the main active component in the study cited above. It would seem advisable to utilize *Cinnamomum verum* in order to capture the efficacy without the potential side effects of coumarin. This anti-inflammatory effect with respect to the nervous system would make *Cinnamomum verum* a candidate for use in a wide variety of conditions associated with neurological inflammation.

Exciting evidence coming from research based on a cellular model of Parkinson's disease demonstrated the possible utility of cinnamon with respect to this neurodegenerative disease.[3] Cinnamaldehyde was able to provide protection against hydrogen peroxide in the cellular model of the disease. It would be wise to incorporate *Cinnamomum verum* into the diet of persons attempting to prevent Parkinson's disease. It may also be beneficial in preventing further progression of damage to the dopaminergic cells after the process has already commenced. Again, the use of the *verum* species maximizes efficacy and minimizes side effects by avoiding the coumarin while providing the cinnamaldehyde.

In Alzheimer's disease, cinnamon appears to be a promising option for prevention and treatment through the prevention of the aggregation of tau protein, the prevention of beta-amyloid aggregation, and through anti-neuroinflammatory and neuroprotective activity.[4-5] Cinnamon may also be beneficial in Alzheimer's treatment and prevention through its antioxidant effects, effects on insulin resistance and blood sugar, and the prevention of neurotoxicity from beta-amyloid.[6-7]

In summary, the use of cinnamon should be considered as a component of a healthy plant-based diet for the prevention and treatment of a variety of neurological conditions. In amounts typically used in food, when the *verum* species is utilized, the safety profile should be excellent. This herb has strong potential for providing beneficial effects in Alzheimer's disease, Parkinson's disease, and multiple sclerosis. It should also be considered in other neurological conditions, particularly neurodegenerative diseases, which may benefit from cinnamon's anti-oxidant, anti-inflammatory, and neuroprotective effects.

Crocus sativus (SAFFRON)

Saffron is a spice harvested from the flowers of *Crocus sativus*, and it has great value in the practice of herbal neurology. This spice has significant effects on the nervous system. There is evidence supporting saffron's effectiveness in treating depression.[1-2] In addition, saffron should be considered a strong candidate for inclusion in a comprehensive treatment protocol for Alzheimer's disease. The evidence suggests that saffron is both safe and effective for Alzheimer's disease.[2-5] Interestingly, the plant also has anti-inflammatory, antioxidant, and anti-convulsant effects. Based on the review of this evidence, this spice should be considered for incorporation into the diet as a general preventative measure to maintain neurological and psychiatric health. With respect to treatment, it certainly deserves high regard in terms of its ability to address depression and Alzheimer's disease. In general, the dosages utilized are between 30-50 mg per day.[6] Dosages under 1500 mg per day are considered non-toxic. Even with lower doses, minor side effects are possible, such as dry mouth, nausea, and dizziness. The literature advises caution in patients with renal insufficiency or those on anticoagulant therapy. Only use small culinary dosages during pregnancy.[7-8] Drug interactions may occur with anti-hypertensive drugs.[9]

Cuminum cyminum (CUMIN)

Cumin may be useful in the prevention of Parkinson's disease.[1] In addition, cumin could potentially be utilized as an anti-inflammatory agent, which would have broad implications in neurology.[2] It would seem wise to incorporate this spice into one's diet in amounts typically used for food preparation. The spice is generally safe, but medication interactions could occur in patients taking diabetic medications (cumin may lower blood glucose), anti-coagulants (cumin may have anti-coagulant effects), or rifampin (cumin may increase absorption of the drug).[3] It may also be prudent to not utilize cumin for two weeks prior to surgery. Its safety is unknown in pregnancy and breast-feeding.

Curcuma longa (TURMERIC)

Turmeric is a spice that has thousands of years of use. It is an important plant in the Ayurvedic system of medicine. The evidence supporting the use of turmeric in the prevention and treatment of Alzheimer's disease is strong enough to support its usage as part of a treatment plan.[1-6] Potential mechanisms of action include metal chelating and antioxidant and anti-inflammatory properties. In addition, turmeric has profound activity against beta-amyloid. It should be noted that infections are well-known as being a potential cause of neurological and psychiatric disorders (syphilis, Lyme disease, etc.). Turmeric has antiviral, antibacterial, anti-fungal, and anti-parasitic properties which may play a role in terms of the plant's positive effect on neurological disorders.

Turmeric should be utilized as part of the prevention and treatment strategy for Parkinson's disease.[4-7] There is evidence suggesting that such a strategy may prove useful with respect to this neurodegenerative disease. In addition, there is evidence supporting the use of turmeric for the prevention and treatment of multiple sclerosis.[6,8-9] Turmeric should also be considered for use in the prevention and treatment of neurological damage from heavy metals, diabetic encephalopathy, amyotrophic lateral sclerosis, traumatic brain injury, glaucoma, Down syndrome, and age-related macular degeneration. Turmeric also has evidence supporting its use in pain relief.[10] It can also be considered for use in COVID-19-related issues.[11]

It is obvious that this plant should form a critical component of a total prevention and treatment program for numerous neurological conditions. Dosage, administration, side effects, contraindications, and other issues should be considered.[12-16] It is strongly recommended that whole turmeric be utilized. Using isolated curcumin is not recommended; it may be less effective with more potential for side effects. The best way to incorporate turmeric is as a spice added to a healthy plant-based diet. A small amount of black pepper should be used with the turmeric to increase the effectiveness. Having this turmeric/black pepper combination with a healthy whole-plant source of fat (such as raw avocado or raw walnuts) should maximize the positive effects of turmeric. Absorption could potentially be increased with the simultaneous consumption of pineapple (for the bromelain). The benefits to overall health from turmeric consumption are broad-based and research supports the usage of this plant in the general population. Contradictory information exists on the safety of turmeric in pregnancy, so caution is advised. People should be cautious of using turmeric if they have gastric ulcers or gallstones.

Turmeric triggers bile release and probably would be useful in the prevention of stones. If the stones are already present, turmeric use could be harmful. Excessive turmeric may increase the risk of kidney stones in those prone to the condition. There are numerous drug interactions.[17]

Recommended dosages vary widely. By weight, there are recommendations ranging from 1-9 grams per day. By volume, dosage recommendations vary from ¼ teaspoon to almost 2 tablespoons per day. It would seem wise to be conservative for general preventative purposes, and thus ¼ teaspoon per day should be utilized as a general neurological preventative, along with black pepper and some whole plant-based fat (almonds, walnuts, avocado, etc.). The plant's safety profile is good throughout the ranges discussed above. However, long historical safety information based on food usage is limited to 1 teaspoon per day. Perhaps this higher dosage of 1 teaspoon should be utilized in active treatment protocols, with the lower ¼ teaspoon dosage reserved for prevention.

To avoid any potential heavy metal contamination with turmeric (and all spices), please source your spices from reputable suppliers (or grow your own). Preference should be given to organic suppliers with high quality-control standards. This quality control issue cannot be emphasized enough, as heavy metal contamination (which can be used deliberately in the case of turmeric in order to change its color) is to be absolutely avoided by everyone, particularly those concerned with neurological health.

Ginkgo biloba (GINKGO)

This plant should be strongly considered for use in herbal neurology. *Ginkgo biloba* may be helpful in the prevention and treatment of cerebral vascular spasms.[1] In addition, the plant may be useful in acute ischemic stroke treatment.[2] This herb may also have utility in the treatment of migraine headaches.[3] Ginkgo biloba is likely to be helpful in the treatment of tardive syndromes[4] and should be strongly considered for the treatment of schizophrenia,[5] as well as for the treatment of Huntington's disease.[6] Very limited evidence suggests that the plant could be helpful in autism treatment.[7] *Ginkgo biloba* should be strongly considered for the treatment of Alzheimer's disease.[8-10] In fact, the plant should be considered in the treatment of vascular dementia, Alzheimer's disease, mixed dementia, and mild cognitive impairment.[11] In treating the dizziness and tinnitus associated with dementia, this herb appears to be effective.[12] Thus, this plant should receive strong consideration for broad use in neurology.

Dosage, safety, and other issues related to the plant must be considered.[13-16] There is a risk of allergy due to ginkgolic acid when the crude leaves are utilized. *Gingko biloba* is a plant where some processing may decrease side effects and increase efficacy. However, my general position is that the use of whole plants, whenever possible, is preferable. The wisdom inherent in nature tends to be better represented in preparations using the whole plant (or whatever part of the plant has medicinal value). Sometimes the short-term benefits from an herbal extract may come at the cost of long-term side effects, which can often be avoided by utilizing whole preparations. In fact, this same ginkgolic acid, whose exposure through crude leaf usage is of concern, appears to have anti-cancer effects.[17] Whether one chooses to use a whole leaf preparation or an extract, a high-quality organic source for the plant material is strongly recommended. While 120 mg per day of the extract is a common dosage, for maximum efficacy, a higher dosage (240 mg of the extract) is suggested. If utilizing a whole-leaf preparation, follow the manufacturer's suggestion for dosage. The safety profile is good. Avoid using ginkgo with other anti-coagulants. Avoid use in pregnancy and in hemophilia. Headaches and gastrointestinal side effects may occur. Effects on the menstrual cycle, including anovulation may occur.

Hericium erinaceus (LION'S MANE)

Hericium erinaceus, also called Lion's Mane, is an edible mushroom. The mushroom consists of the mycelium and the fruiting body. The fruiting body is used for culinary and medical purposes,[1] and the mycelium is the subject of significant interest in the field of neurology.[2] The fruiting body may be helpful in treating mild cognitive impairment. The mycelium may be useful in the prevention and treatment of Alzheimer's disease and Parkinson's disease. It may also be helpful in treating depression. Utility in terms of treating ischemic stroke is also possible. The mycelium should be considered to potentially improve nerve regeneration.

The safety of the fruiting body should be excellent due to not only the medical-use data but particularly due to its safe culinary use. The mycelium also has an outstanding safety profile. Either follow the manufacturer's instructions on dosage or consume it in normal food quantities. For maximum safety, use it as a culinary mushroom only, particularly in pregnancy and breastfeeding. This will help minimize any potential safety issues, including possible drug interactions. This mushroom appears to have an interesting role in neurology and should form part of the diet of people who wish to prevent or treat various neurological conditions.

Hypericum perforatum (ST. JOHN'S WORT)

Hypericum perforatum, also known as St. John's Wort, deserves consideration for use in herbal neurological medicine. There is very strong evidence supporting its use in mild to moderate depression.[1-3] Efficacy in severe depression is questionable, according to the scientific literature. This herb can be utilized in pain management,[4] and should be considered for use in premenstrual dysphoric disorder.[5] *Hypericum perforatum* should be strongly considered for use in all neurodegenerative diseases, and there is particularly strong evidence for its potential benefits in Parkinson's disease and Alzheimer's disease.[6] The potential neuroprotective and antioxidant effects are only one justification for such use. The plant's potential to reduce inflammation in the nervous system would also make it highly useful in such situations. In addition, the antiviral, antibacterial, and anti-fungal effects of the herb may further improve the efficacy of the plant in neurological disorders. Taken together, the plant should be considered foundational for the herbal treatment of neurological disorders such as Alzheimer's disease, Parkinson's disease, multiple sclerosis, and amyotrophic lateral sclerosis. The herb is suggested to be potentially helpful with insomnia, anxiety, and nerve damage.[7-8]

Dosage, side effects, contraindications, and other issues should be considered.[6-11] The plant is very safe in general. Side effects are rare, but may include photo-toxicity, allergic reactions, headaches, gastrointestinal symptoms, dry mouth, etc. Avoid in pregnancy. Drug interactions are numerous. As the plant affects liver enzymes, numerous categories of drugs will be affected, generally causing reduced levels of these drugs in the body (faster clearance). An experienced healthcare practitioner must evaluate all drugs that the patient may be taking and make an appropriate decision on a case-by-case basis. In addition, caution must be advised with respect to using *Hypericum perforatum* simultaneously with selective serotonin re-uptake inhibitors (SSRIs) or mono-amine oxidase (MAO) inhibitors. Such combinations may be dangerous. Dosage for infusions of the herb can be 1 teaspoon dried herb in 1 cup boiling water three times per day. The herb should infuse for 10 minutes (maximum 15 minutes). The whole herb can be utilized in total daily dosages of 1.5 to 6 grams. Standardized extracts should be used in lower dosages, generally from 900 mg to 1200 mg total per day. In all cases, split the total daily dosage into 3 equal dosages throughout the day. Manufacturer's instructions will be helpful for various products such as tinctures, etc. The preference is for whole herb usage as opposed to standardized extracts. This author recommends using an organic, ecological, sustainable source that utilizes the whole plant.

Nepeta cataria (CATNIP, CATMINT)

This plant is commonly known as catnip or catmint. It has a place in neurology. However, such use is based more on tradition and experience than modern scientific literature. This author has elected to include the herb because of personal experience demonstrating its effectiveness in relieving muscle spasticity in a neurological disorder. While there is little in the modern scientific literature on this plant in terms of neurological conditions, traditional herbalism considers the plant to be helpful with anxiety, insomnia, convulsions/epilepsy, and muscle spasms.[1-5] The herb has a strong safety profile, including when utilized in children. Excessive use should be avoided due to nausea and vomiting. Avoid use in pregnancy. The dosage for an infusion can be 2 teaspoons of the dried herb in 1 cup of boiling water.[6] Infusion time can be 10-15 minutes. Adults can consume 1 cup up to 3 times per day. Children's dosage should be adjusted based on their weight/age. In other forms, follow the manufacturer's instructions. In my opinion, despite the lack of scientific literature, this plant holds an important place in neurological herbal medicine.

Nigella sativa (BLACK CARAWAY, BLACK CUMIN)

This plant has a profoundly broad range of uses in herbal medicine and also in herbal neurology. In English-speaking societies, it is sometimes referred to as black caraway or black cumin. The plant has antiviral, antibacterial, anti-parasitic, and anti-fungal effects.[1] This makes the plant potentially useful for infections which may play a role in neurological symptoms. The plant may protect against neurological toxicity from the effects of various toxins, including aluminum, lead, ethanol, gentamicin, and toluene.[2] This herb may be useful in treating anxiety, depression, Alzheimer's disease, Parkinson's disease, multiple sclerosis, epilepsy, neuropathic pain, and neurological trauma.[3] It may also have beneficial effects on memory and learning and may potentially be useful in stroke and drug addiction recovery (opiate withdrawal). *Nigella sativa* should also be considered for possible treatment of any condition with nervous system inflammation and for schizophrenia.[4] It should also be noted that this plant may be useful for treating COVID-19-related issues.[5] Outside the realm of neurology, the herb may be beneficial in the treatment of elevated cholesterol, diabetes, hypertension, cancer, asthma, ulcers due to *Helicobacter pylori*, obesity, HIV infection, and male infertility.[6-8] In fact, the scientific literature is so extensive and broad-based that it seems that the herb could potentially be utilized for a very large list of potential diseases. Dosages of the whole seed (powdered) vary but range between 500 mg per day up to 3,000 mg per day in adults. Dosages in children should be adjusted according to age and weight. For example, for treatment of parasites in children, the literature suggests 40 mg/kg in a single dosage of the powdered seed. The safety profile is excellent as long as reasonable dosages (as described above) are used. The herb may not be safe at dosages above those typically used in food during pregnancy.[9] It would be wise to avoid use prior to surgery as a precaution. Some adverse digestive symptoms may occur with treatment (bloating, nausea, etc.), however, this is more likely to occur when ingesting the oil rather than the whole seed.

I generally recommend using the whole seed (ground) instead of the oil preparation. However, the oil form definitely has a place in medicine. My preference is generally to avoid oils when the whole form of a plant can be utilized. Mild changes in kidney and liver markers may occur with both the seeds and the oil. Interactions are possible with numerous drugs. In summation, *Nigella sativa* should be considered profoundly useful in the application of herbal medicine in neurology.

Passiflora spp. (PASSIONFLOWER)

Commonly referred to as passionflower, different species within this genus are utilized, although most commonly *Passiflora incarnata* is used. Passionflower may have utility in the treatment of alcoholism and nicotine addiction.[1] In acute menopausal syndrome, it also appears to have efficacy.[2] The plant can be useful in the treatment of insomnia, anxiety, and irritability, and has antiviral, anti-inflammatory, sedative, anti-asthmatic, anti-tussive, anti-diabetic, antioxidant, and anticancer properties.[3-7] The plant should also be considered for use in epilepsy, muscle spasms, spasticity, and potentially for symptomatic relief in multiple sclerosis and Parkinson's disease.[8-11]

The plant has an excellent safety profile. It should not be used during pregnancy. Caution should be advised with possible drug interactions, particularly with substances with overlapping functions, such as barbiturates, sedatives, benzodiazepines, etc. The dosage can be 1 cup of tea (1 teaspoon dried herb per cup boiling water) at night for insomnia. 1 cup twice per day (1 teaspoon dried herb per cup boiling water) can be utilized for anxiety. Infusion time should be 15 minutes for both of these uses. The dried herb itself can be consumed at 1/4 gram to 2 grams up to three times per day orally.[12] For other preparations, follow the manufacturer's instructions. Although generally safe when used at recommended dosages, side effects are possible, including confusion, drowsiness, dizziness, and liver and pancreatic toxicity. In general, this plant holds a very important place in neurological medicine.

Phyllanthus emblica (INDIAN GOOSEBERRY, AMLA, AMALAKI)

This plant, also referred to as Indian Gooseberry, Amla, Amalaki, or *Emblica officinalis*, has a remarkable value in herbal medicine. The berries are the part most commonly utilized. The plant has many properties associated with it, including anti-fungal, antibacterial, antiviral, anti-ulcer, antioxidant, anticancer, immunomodulatory, anti-inflammatory, anti-atherogenic, pain-relieving, antipyretic, anti-tussive, nephroprotective, hepato-protective, and neuroprotective effects.[1-2] For cholesterol reduction and for cancer prevention and treatment, this plant should be strongly considered.[3-4] Its safety profile is excellent. The dry powder can be utilized at 2 grams twice per day. Drug interactions are possible because the herb can lower blood sugar and have anticoagulant effects. Caution is advised with people utilizing the herb along with drugs with such effects. It may be advisable to not utilize amla prior to and immediately after surgery due to its anti-coagulant effects. People with bleeding disorders should be cautious about using amla berry. With all of these considerations in mind, I believe that amla has a profound place in herbal medicine, including herbal neurology. It should also be considered for general health promotion. The incredibly broad range of action of this plant, including the neuroprotective effects, make it a strong candidate for use in neurological conditions. Through direct and indirect mechanisms, it has a strong potential to improve health.

Piper methysticum (KAVA, KAVA KAVA)

Kava is a plant that may have uses in neurology/psychiatry. It should be considered for use in the treatment of anxiety, and it may also have neuroprotective, anesthetic, sedative, and anticonvulsant effects.[1-3] The plant may also be useful as an anti-spasmodic in neurological disorders, and its safety is generally good, with a few important caveats.[4-7] People with depression should be cautious about its use. It may be helpful with insomnia. Those with Parkinson's disease should not use this plant. Pregnant and breastfeeding women should also not use kava. Those with liver disease or alcoholism should avoid kava. In addition, large doses and prolonged use of kava without breaks should be avoided. Negative effects on the liver are possible, and dermatological side effects are also possible. Avoid combining it with drugs with similar effects, such as sedatives, benzodiazepines, etc. There are numerous potential drug interactions. Kava may impair one's ability to drive safely, and thus, the highest level of caution is advised. Use of kava should be stopped prior to surgery.[8]

Dosage is variable, depending on the method of administration and whether you're using whole versus extract, etc. For a simple tea, 1 teaspoon of the root (sliced and dried) should be lightly simmered for ten minutes (1 cup of water per 1 teaspoon of root). After straining, up to 2 cups per day can be drunk. For other preparations, follow specific dosages provided with the products. The whole root form may be utilized in 1 gram dosages (as needed). Avoid using high dosages (for example, above 9 grams per day can affect liver function). Stay at the lowest dosage possible for the shortest period of time necessary. This herb should be utilized for short-term purposes until the underlying cause of the problem can be addressed. The herb can be used socially, occasionally, or for short-term symptomatic relief, and traditional use of the herb must be respected. Liver toxicity may be more connected to using the stems or leaves rather than the root of the plant.[9] Therefore for maximum safety, only the root should be utilized. Regardless, liver enzymes should be checked regularly in those using kava for more than

28 days. In summation, this plant can be utilized in herbal neurology, but use should be short-term. This is not a foundational herbal treatment for neurological disorders, but rather an interim herb for relief of specific symptoms. A comprehensive, "treat the cause" approach should always be taken with any disease.

Punica granatum (POMEGRANATE)

Although in herbal medicine, leaves, roots, bark, flowers, seeds, and fruit from the pomegranate may be utilized, for food, one typically consumes the arils and seeds. The arils are the outer red covering around the seeds. I recommend using both the seeds and the arils, in line with a more whole-plant philosophy. Consumption of the aril-seed combination may be beneficial in prevention and treatment of cardiovascular disease and hypertension, and this is of profound importance to neurological issues since a healthy vascular system has a significant impact on the brain.[1] Ingestion of the aril-seed combination may also be beneficial in the prevention and treatment of Alzheimer's disease. The arils have both antiinflammatory and antioxidant effects, and this would make them beneficial in a wide variety of neurological conditions. Interestingly, consumption of the arils may have neuroprotective effects and has the potential to help prevent the brain damage seen in neonatal hypoxic-ischemic brain injury.[2] Ingestion of both the arils and seeds also appears to have anticancer effects. In traditional herbal medicine, the bark is typically used against parasites, particularly tapeworm.[3-5] Parasitic infection can lead to neurological complications, and so this property of bark may prove useful in herbal neurology. The safety of the arils and seeds is excellent; however, other parts of the plant require caution.[6] Upset stomach, dizziness, and muscle cramps may occur with the use of the root bark. For maximum safety, use only the arils and seeds. There are numerous potential drug interactions, so caution is advised. Pregnant and breastfeeding women should only utilize the arils/seeds in normal food quantities and avoid other types of preparations (concentrated extracts, root, stem, and rind products, for example). If used for neurological conditions, it is recommended that the arils and seeds be incorporated into a healthy plant-based diet. Pomegranate aril and seed consumption should be encouraged in a wide variety of neurological conditions, for both preventative and treatment purposes.

Rosmarinus officinalis (ROSEMARY)

Rosemary is an herb commonly utilized in food preparation. The herb has neuroprotective effects.[1] Rosemary may reduce cognitive deficits and has anticancer, antioxidant, and anti-diabetic properties. The herb also possesses anti-inflammatory effects. Rosemary has the potential to be beneficial in the prevention and treatment of Alzheimer's disease, Parkinson's disease, and depression.[2] Further, this herb may have utility in the treatment of myasthenia gravis.[3] Many other issues associated with rosemary must be considered, including other potential uses, dosage, side effects, contraindications, etc.[4-9] Rosemary may be helpful for use as an antiseptic and for treatment of indigestion and flatulence.

Dosage varies depending on the preparation, so follow the manufacturer's instructions. For ground rosemary, up to 1.5 grams may be used 3 times per day. This dosage refers only to the whole herb, not extracts. For tea, 1 teaspoon of dried rosemary per cup of boiling water is used as an infusion. After pouring the boiling water on the herb and covering it, allow 10 or 15 minutes of infusion time. Up to three cups per day can be used. The herb is generally extremely safe, particularly when used in normal food amounts.

In pregnancy, only normal food quantities are permissible. Do not utilize higher dosages in pregnancy. Avoid use in seizures. Large dosages can cause side effects including digestive symptoms and kidney damage. Caution is advised in using rosemary in persons suffering from bleeding disorders. There are numerous potential drug interactions, although all of these are either minor or moderate in severity. Regardless, caution is always advised, and potential interactions should be thoroughly checked. Essentially, rosemary has broad potential for use in herbal neurology but should not be utilized in epilepsy.

Scutellaria baicalensis (HUANG QIN, BAIKAL SKULLCAP, SCUTE ROOT) and *Scutellaria lateriflora* (BLUE SKULLCAP)

Scutellaria baicalensis should be considered for use in herbal neurology. The plant is neuroprotective, potentially helpful in preventing and treating Alzheimer's disease and Parkinson's disease, and has anti-inflammatory, antioxidant, anti-anxiety, anti-convulsant, sedative, cognitive-enhancing, and neuro-regenerative properties.[1] The plant may also have potential use in traumatic brain injury.[2] In addition, *Scutellaria baicalensis* may have utility in cerebral ischemia and stroke.[3] This herb is remarkable in that it has the potential to stimulate neurogenesis.[4] Its safety profile is very good, although certain issues need to be considered, including other possible uses of the herb, dosage, etc.[5-6] In general, the herb is very safe, although drowsiness may occur. There are numerous potential drug interactions. Avoid use prior to surgery. Caution is advised in patients with bleeding disorders, those taking anti-coagulants, anti-diabetic medications, anti-hypertensive medications, and estrogen. Those with estrogen-sensitive conditions such as ovarian, breast, or uterine cancer should exercise caution. The herb has potential utility outside of neurology, including for hepatitis and lung infections. In Traditional Chinese Medicine, it may be utilized for allergies, and herbalists may find it is also helpful for asthma. Follow the manufacturer's instructions for dosage. But generally, the dried powder can be utilized at a dosage of 3-10 grams daily. More concentrated products or extracts obviously should be used in lower amounts. This herb should be strongly considered for numerous neurological conditions. It has profoundly broad potential for use. It is of the highest value in herbal neurology.

Scutellaria lateriflora should be considered for use in treating epilepsy and anxiety.[7] Herbalists consider the plant to potentially have a place in the treatment of insomnia, hydrophobia, muscle spasticity, schizophrenia, neuralgia, chorea, and drug addiction withdrawal.[8-11] This plant is very safe, however, there are some considerations.[12] Avoid use prior to surgery and be cautious in terms of combining with other sedatives (potential additive effects). Side effects generally should not occur when using normal dosages. Follow the manufacturer's instructions for specific products. Infusions can be made with 1-2 teaspoons of herb (dried) per cup of boiling water. After pouring the water on the herb, allow 10 or 15 minutes of infusion time. Up to 3 cups per day can be ingested. Overdose of the herb in tincture form can cause serious neurological side effects, including twitching and confusion. Overall, this plant deserves the highest regard in terms of its utility in herbal neurology.

Based on my personal experience, the plant may be remarkably effective in easing muscle spasticity, difficulty in walking, and muscle coordination issues associated with neurological dysfunction. I believe

that the plant should be strongly considered for use in multiple sclerosis, epilepsy, Parkinson's disease, and other neurological/psychiatric
situations.

Syzygium aromaticum (CLOVE)

Clove has anti-inflammatory, antioxidant, antibacterial, anti-fungal,
and anesthetic properties.[1-3] The spice also has antiviral activity.[4] Other
potential uses, dosage, and safety should be considered.[5-9] Herbalists
may also use clove for nausea and flatulence, while clove oil may be
used for dental issues and pain relief. Cloves may have anti-parasitic
properties. The spice, when used in normal quantities in food, is safe.
Excessive quantities can cause irritation or even damage tissue in the
mouth.

Clove oil has a higher risk of side effects, particularly when consumed internally. In children, consumption of the oil can cause fluid
imbalance, seizures, and liver damage. Applying clove oil topically is
generally safe, although irritation can occur. Excessive application of
the oil for dental purposes can damage tissues. It is recommended to
dilute clove essential oil before utilizing it for topical purposes. Avoid
cloves prior to surgery and exercise caution if using anti-coagulants or
in patients with bleeding disorders. Infusions of clove can be made by
pouring 1 cup of boiling water on some cloves and allowing 10 minutes
infusion time before consumption.

I suggest simply incorporating cloves as a spice in normal food
quantities. Follow the manufacturer's instructions for other clove preparations. Overall, it seems wise to incorporate this spice into the diet for
prevention and treatment of neurological disorders, as the antioxidant
and anti-inflammatory effects may be beneficial. The antibacterial and

anti-fungal properties may also contribute indirectly to neurological health, due to the potential neurological effects of infectious diseases.

Vaccinium myrtillus (BILBERRIES)

Bilberries are edible berries closely related to blueberries (of which there are numerous species in the *Vaccinium* genus). Bilberries have antioxidant and anti-inflammatory effects and may improve cognitive and neurological function.[1] They may also be beneficial to cardiovascular and ocular health.

Safety, dosage, contraindications, and other potential uses should be considered.[2-7] Bilberries may be helpful in treating retinopathy, chronic venous insufficiency, dysmenorrhea, rheumatoid arthritis, diarrhea, glaucoma, eye strain, varicose veins, and myopia. They may also be beneficial in treating multiple sclerosis through potentially positive effects on the blood-brain barrier. The safety profile is excellent. When eating the berries, there should be no side effects or safety issues. Long-term use of the leaves is not recommended due to possible kidney damage. Thus, the information and recommendations here apply only to the use of berries. Bilberries may potentiate anti-coagulant therapy, so caution is advised. In terms of dosage, the berries can be eaten as desired. Follow manufacturer's dosage instructions if taking another form of bilberry preparation made from the berries. A dosage of 20 grams up to 60 grams per day of dried bilberries is suggested. It should be noted that blueberries are essentially considered interchangeable with bilberries in terms of beneficial effects.

One suggested dosage for blueberries in multiple sclerosis is up to 2 pounds per week of frozen blueberries (divide this amount throughout the week). Blueberries may lower blood sugar, and thus those with diabetes and those taking anti-diabetic drugs should be cautious when taking blueberries.[8] Again, as with bilberries, avoid using the blueberry leaf. Use the berries only. There is evidence specific to blueberries demonstrating efficacy in terms of treating age-related memory loss. However, one would expect bilberries to have similar effects. Overall, it seems wise to recommend that bilberries and blueberries be incorporated into the diet of anyone concerned about preventing and treating numerous neurological disorders. In particular, memory-related issues and multiple sclerosis receive a high recommendation for use.

Valeriana officinalis (VALERIAN)

Valerian has a place in the practice of herbal neurology. The herb has sedative effects and is useful in treating insomnia.[1] It may be helpful in attention deficit hyperactivity disorder[2] and in treating fatigue and sleep disturbances associated with multiple sclerosis.[3] Other issues, potential uses, safety, contraindications, and dosage need to be considered.[4-13] Valerian can be useful in treating hot flashes associated with menopause and may be helpful with premenstrual syndrome. It may be helpful with anxiety, epilepsy, posttraumatic stress disorder, heart arrhythmia, depression, and muscle spasms. Infusions can be made by pouring 1 cup boiling water on 1 teaspoon of dried root and allowing 10 minutes of infusion time. The powdered root can be taken in vegan capsules at a dosage of up to 1000 mg. Take this dosage about 30 minutes prior to sleeping in cases of insomnia. For non-insomnia uses, 500 mg to 1000 mg of the powdered root in vegan capsules can be taken four times per day (lower dosages and fewer times per day are also acceptable). For other valerian products, follow the manufacturer's instructions.

Valerian root is generally safe when used in normal dosages. Upset stomach is a possible side effect in some people. It can have paradoxical stimulating effects in some individuals. Headaches, uneasiness, and morning drowsiness are some additional possible side effects. It should not be used by pregnant women. Avoid use with alcohol, sedatives, benzodiazepines, barbiturates, central nervous system depressants, sleep aids, etc. There are numerous potential drug interactions. Avoid use prior to surgery. Caution is advised in terms of driving while utilizing valerian root. Avoid using large dosages for long periods of time. Under such circumstances, it is possible to experience valerian withdrawal syndrome. To avoid this syndrome, it is wise to slowly decrease the dosage in order to safely come off the herb. Overdoses of valerian can cause hallucinations, headaches, and spasms, among other symptoms.

In general, it can be said that valerian root should be considered for use in herbal neurology under certain circumstances. It is preferable that such use be short-term and for symptomatic relief and that other therapies (herbs, plant-based nutrition, etc.) be utilized to address neurological conditions on a long-term basis.

Zingiber officinale (GINGER)

Ginger should be considered for use in herbal neurology. The herb has neuroprotective and anti-inflammatory properties and may be useful in the treatment of multiple sclerosis.[1] Further, ginger has antioxidant and immunomodulatory properties, further increasing the likelihood of positive effects in the treatment of multiple sclerosis.[2] Through effects on nuclear transcription factor kappa B, ginger may be helpful in the prevention and treatment of Alzheimer's disease and multiple

sclerosis.[3] In addition, ginger has anti-fungal, anticancer, antibacterial, anti-diabetic, anti-ulcer, anti-emetic, hepato-protective, and
migraine-relieving effects.[4] The plant may be useful in the treatment of
age-related neurological disorders.[5] Safety, dosage, contraindications,
and other potential uses should be considered.[6-13] Ginger may have anti-
spasmodic, antiviral, and antipyretic effects. The plant can improve
circulation. It may be useful for motion sickness. The dosage of ginger
powder (dried) can be 500 mg to 1500 mg up to 3 times daily.

Ginger tea can be utilized up to 2 cups daily. The tea can be
made with a decoction of fresh ginger or an infusion of powdered
ginger. For the decoction, use 1 teaspoon per cup of boiling water,
simmer for 10 minutes, and strain. For the infusion, pour 1 cup of
boiling water on ½ teaspoon ginger (powder). Infusion time should
be 10 minutes. Only the liquid should be drunk, after separating the
powder from the liquid. For other preparations, follow the manufacturer's instructions.

Caution is advised, as ginger may improve drug absorption. There
are numerous potential drug interactions. In particular, anti-coagulant
drugs and anti-diabetic drugs may have their effects potentiated by
ginger, and thus caution is advised. Digestive discomfort may occur. Side
effects may include heartburn and diarrhea. Menstrual bleeding may
increase in women. Other side effects are possible, particularly if the
dosage is excessive. Persons with gallstones should not utilize ginger at
medicinal dosages. Exercise caution if a patient has bleeding disorders
or diabetes. There are contradictory beliefs on the safety of ginger in
pregnancy. It does appear to be reasonably safe for treating morning
sickness. If utilized in pregnancy, avoid high doses and use the lowest
possible dosage. Dosages of 1 to 6 grams daily of ginger (powdered) for
morning sickness is a general guideline. Overall, ginger appears to have

a strong place in herbal neurology. It should especially be considered for Alzheimer's disease and multiple sclerosis, but its use should not be limited to these neurological issues.

A NOTE ON REFERENCES
THROUGHOUT THIS WORK

It is my firm belief that animal research on sentient forms of life is unethical. Therefore, I have attempted to avoid utilizing and citing references based on direct animal research. This is deliberately done to discourage future research based on animal models, as researchers will be less likely to participate in such experiments if they believe that their work will not be cited. Review articles may be cited that discuss animal research, however, no citation based on direct animal research has been cited intentionally. It is hoped that in vitro, human research, computer models, epidemiological, and other forms of human clinical research will eliminate and replace animal testing/research. The ethics of research require consent, and this clearly cannot occur with animal research.

This project is based on my thesis project through Dominion Herbal College:

Srour, SJ. *The Application of Herbal Medicine in Neurology*. Master Herbalist Thesis. 2019.

It has been significantly expanded into something much broader. Nevertheless, it is important to note that the thesis served as the foundation for this work.

CHAPTER 1 REFERENCES

Allium sativum:

1. Tillotson, AK, NH Tillotson, and R Abel. *The One Earth Herbal Sourcebook: Everything You Need to Know about Chinese, Western, and Ayurvedic Herbal Treatments.* New York, NY: Twin Streams; 2001.

2. Kannappan, R, SC Gupta, JH. Kim, S Reuter, and B. Aggarwal. "Neuro-protection by Spice-Derived Nutraceuticals: You Are What You Eat!" *Molecular Neurobiology.* 2011;44(2):142-159. Doi: 10.1007/ s12035-011-8168-2.

3. Lau, K-K, Y-H Chan, Y-K Wong, et al. "Garlic intake is an independent predictor of endothelial function in patients with ischemic stroke." *The Journal of Nutrition, Health & Aging.* 2013; 17(7): 600-604. Doi: 10.1007/ s12603-013-0043-6.

4. Zhu, Y, R Anand, X Geng, and Y Ding. "A mini review: garlic extract and vascular diseases." *Neurological Research.* 2018; 40(6): 421-425. Doi: 10.1080/01616412.2018.1451269.

5. Ray, B, NB Chauhan, and DK Lahiri. "The 'Aged Garlic Extract' (AGE) and One of its Active Ingredients S-Allyl-LCysteine (SAC) as Potential Preventive and Therapeutic Agents for Alzheimer's Disease (AD)." *Current Medicinal Chemistry.* 2011; 18(22): 3306-3313. Doi: 10.2174/ 092986711796504664.

6. Easley, T, and SH Horne. *The Modern Herbal Dispensatory: a Medicine-Making Guide.* Berkeley, CA: North Atlantic Books; 2016.

7. Hoffmann, D. *The New Holistic Herbal.* Shaftesbury, Dorset: Element; 1994.

8. Balick, MJ, and A Weil. *Rodale's 21st-Century Herbal: a Practical Guide for Healthy Living Using Nature's Most Powerful Plants.* New York, NY: Rodale; 2014.

9. "Garlic Effectiveness, Safety, and Drug Interactions." *RxList.* https://www.rxlist.com/garlic/supplements.htm. Accessed January 15, 2019.

Bacopa monnieri:

1. Shinomol, GK, Muralidhara, MM Bharath. "Exploring the Role of 'Brahmi' (*Bacopa monnieri* and *Centella asiatica*) in Brain Function and Therapy." *Recent Patents on Endocrine, Metabolic & Immune Drug Discovery.* 2011; 5(1): 33-49. Doi: 10.2174/187221411794351833.

2. Cicero, AF, F Fogacci, and M Banach. "Botanicals and phytochemicals active on cognitive decline: The clinical evidence." *Pharmacological Research*. 2018; 130: 204-212. Doi: 10.1016/j.phrs.2017.12.029.

3. Nemetchek, MD, AA Stierle, DB Stierle, and DI Lurie. "The Ayurvedic plant Bacopa monnieri inhibits inflammatory pathways in the brain." *Journal of Ethnopharmacology*. 2017; 197: 92-100. Doi: 10.1016/ j.jep.2016.07.073.

4. Kean, JD, LA Downey, and C Stough. "A systematic review of the Ayurvedic medicinal herb *Bacopa monnieri* in child and adolescent populations." *Complementary Therapies in Medicine*. 2016: 29: 56-62. Doi: 10.1016/j.ctim.2016.09.002.

5. Easley, T, and SH Horne. *The Modern Herbal Dispensatory: a Medicine-Making Guide*. Berkeley, CA: North Atlantic Books; 2016.

6. "Brahmi Effectiveness, Safety, and Drug Interactions." *RxList*. https://www.rxlist. com/brahmi/supplements.htm. Accessed January 15, 2019.

Brassica oleracea:

1. Masci, A, R Mattioli, P Costantino, et al. "Neuroprotective Effect of *Brassica oleracea* Sprouts Crude Juice in a Cellular Model of Alzheimer's Disease." *Oxidative Medicine and Cellular Longevity*. 2015: 1-17. Doi: 10.1155/ 2015/781938.

2. Sun, Y, T Yang, L Mao, F Zhang. "Sulforaphane Protects against Brain Diseases: Roles of Cytoprotective Enzymes." *Austin Journal of Cerebrovascular Disease & Stroke*. 2017; 4(1). Doi: 10.26420/austinjcerebrovascdisstroke.2017.1054.

3. Singh, K, SL Connors, EA Macklin, et al. "Sulforaphane treatment of autism spectrum disorder (ASD)." *Proc Natl Acad Sci U S A*. 2014; 111(43): 15550-15555. Doi: 10.1073/ pnas.1416940111.

4. Lynch, R, EL Diggins, SL Connors, et al. "Sulforaphane from Broccoli Reduces Symptoms of Autism: A Follow-up Case Series from a Randomized Double-blind Study." *Global Advances in Health and Medicine*. 2017; 6. Doi: 10.1177/2164957x17735826.

5. Bent, S, B Lawton, T Warren, et al. "Identification of urinary metabolites that correlate with clinical improvements in children with autism treated with sulforaphane from broccoli." *Molecular Autism*. 2018; 9(1). Doi: 10.1186/s13229-018-0218-4.

6. "Cabbage Effectiveness, Safety, and Drug Interactions." *RxList*. https://www.rxlist. com/cabbage/supplements.htm. Accessed January 15, 2019.

Camelia sinensis:

1. Kakuda, T. "Neuroprotective effects of theanine and its preventive effects on cognitive dysfunction." *Pharmacological Research.* 2011; 64(2): 162-168. Doi: 10.1016/j.phrs.2011.03.010.

2. Hayat, K, H Iqbal, U Malik, U Bilal, and S Mushtaq. "Tea and Its Consumption: Benefits and Risks." *Critical Reviews in Food Science and Nutrition.* 2015; 55(7): 939-954. Doi: 10.1080/10408398.2012.678949.

3. Pervin, M, K Unno, T Ohishi, H Tanabe, N Miyoshi, and Y Nakamura. "Beneficial Effects of Green Tea Catechins on Neurodegenerative Diseases." *Molecules.* 2018; 23(6): 1297. Doi: 10.3390/molecules23061297.

4. Morgan, LA, and O Grundmann. "Preclinical and Potential Applications of Common Western Herbal Supplements as Complementary Treatment in Parkinson's Disease." *Journal of Dietary Supplements.* 2017; 14(4): 453-466. Doi: 10.1080/19390211.2016.1263710.

5. Ide, K, N Matsuoka, H Yamada, D Furushima, and K Kawakami. "Effects of Tea Catechins on Alzheimer's Disease: Recent Updates and Perspectives." *Molecules.* 2018; 23(9): 2357. Doi: 10.3390/molecules23092357.

6. Farzaei, MH, Z Shahpiri, R Bahramsoltani, MM Nia, F Najafi, and R Rahimi. "Efficacy and Tolerability of Phytomedicines in Multiple Sclerosis Patients: A Review." *CNS Drugs.* 2017; 31(10): 867-889. Doi: 10.1007/ s40263-017-0466-4.

7. Yu, Y, S Hayashi, X Cai, et al. "Pu-Erh Tea Extract Induces the Degradation of FET Family Proteins Involved in the Pathogenesis of Amyotrophic Lateral Sclerosis." *BioMed Research International.* 2014: 1-12. Doi: 10.1155/ 2014/254680/.

8. Cunha, JP. "Green Tea *(Camellia Sinensis):* Side Effects, Dosages, Treatment, Interactions, Warnings." *RxList.* https://www.rxlist.com/ consumer_green_tea_camellia_sinensis/drugs-condition.htm. Accessed January 15, 2019.

9. Tillotson, AK, NH Tillotson, and R Abel. *The One Earth Herbal Sourcebook: Everything You Need to Know about Chinese, Western, and Ayurvedic Herbal Treatments.* New York, NY: Twin Streams; 2001.

10. Balick, MJ, and A Weil. *Rodale's 21st-Century Herbal: a Practical Guide for Healthy Living Using Nature's Most Powerful Plants.* New York, NY: Rodale; 2014.

Cannabis sativa:

1. Li, H, Y Liu, D Tian, et al. "Overview of cannabidiol (CBD) and its analogues: Structures, biological activities, and neuroprotective mechanisms in epilepsy and Alzheimer's disease." *Eur J Med Chem.* 2020; 192: 112163. Doi: 10.1016/j.ejmech.2020.112163.

2. Peng, J, M Fan, C An, F Ni, W Huang, and J Luo. "A narrative review of molecular mechanism and therapeutic effect of cannabidiol (CBD)." *Basic Clin Pharmacol Toxicol.* 2022; 130(4): 439-456. Doi: 10.1111/bcpt.13710.

3. Bonaccorso, S, A Ricciardi, C Zangani, S Chiappini, and F Schifano. "Cannabidiol (CBD) use in psychiatric disorders: A systematic review." *Neurotoxicology.* 2019; 74: 282-298. Doi: 10.1016/j.neuro.2019.08.002.

4. Elms, L, S Shannon, S Hughes, and N Lewis. "Cannabidiol in the Treatment of Post-Traumatic Stress Disorder: A Case Series." *J Altern Complement Med.* 2019; 25(4): 392-397. Doi: 10.1089/acm.2018.0437

5. Pahr, K. "Beginner's Guide to CBD." *Healthline.* Published August 3, 2018. Accessed August 14, 2023. https://www.healthline.com/health/yourcbd-guide.

Centella asiatica:

1. Chen, C-L, W-H Tsai, C-J Chen, and T-M Pan. "*Centella asiatica* extract protects against amyloid ß1–40 induced neurotoxicity in neuronal cells by activating the antioxidative defence system." *Journal of Traditional and Complementary Medicine.* 2016; 6(4): 362-369. Doi: 10.1016/ j.jtcme.2015.07.002.

2. Hossain, S, M Hashimoto, M Katakura, AA Mamun, and O Shido. "Medicinal value of asiaticoside for Alzheimer's disease as assessed using single-molecule-detection fluorescence correlation spectroscopy, laser-scanning microscopy, transmission electron microscopy, and in silico docking." *BMC Complementary and Alternative Medicine.* 2015; 15(1). Doi: 10.1186/s12906-015-0620-9.

3. Berrocal, R, P Vasudevaraju, SS Indi, KRSS Rao, and K Rao. "In vitro Evidence that an Aqueous Extract of Centella asiatica Modulates α-Synuclein Aggregation Dynamics." *Journal of Alzheimers Disease.* 2014; 39(2): 457-465. Doi: 10.3233/jad-131187.

4. Farhana, KM, RG Malueka, S Wibowo, and A Gofir. "Effectiveness of Gotu Kola Extract 750 mg and 1000 mg Compared with Folic Acid 3 mg in Improving Vascular Cognitive Impairment after Stroke." *Evidence-Based Complementary and Alternative Medicine.* 2016; 2016: 1-6. Doi: 10.1155/2016/2795915.

5. Orhan, IE. *"Centella asiatica (L.)* Urban: From Traditional Medicine to Modern Medicine with Neuroprotective Potential." *Evidence-Based Complementary and Alternative Medicine.* 2012; 2012: 1-8. Doi: 10.1155/2012/946259.

6. Lokanathan, Y, N Omar, NN Ahmed Puzi, A Saim, and R Hj Idrus. "Recent Updates in Neuroprotective and Neuroregenerative Potential of *Centella asiatica.*" *The Malaysian Journal of Medical Sciences.* 2016; 23(1): 4-14.

7. "Gotu Kola Effectiveness, Safety, and Drug Interactions" *RxList.* https://www.rxlist.com/gotu_kola/supplements.htm. Accessed January 15, 2019.

8. Cunha, JP. "Gotu Kola: Uses, Side Effects, Dosage & Drug Interactions." *RxList.* https://www.rxlist.com/consumer_gotu_kola/drugs-condition.htm. Accessed January 15, 2019.

9. Easley, T, and SH Horne. *The Modern Herbal Dispensatory: a Medicine-Making Guide.* Berkeley, CA: North Atlantic Books; 2016.

10. Balick, MJ, and A Weil. *Rodale's 21st-Century Herbal: a Practical Guide for Healthy Living Using Nature's Most Powerful Plants.* New York, NY: Rodale; 2014.

11. Tilgner, S. *Herbal Medicine: from the Heart of the Earth.* Pleasant Hill, OR: Wise Acres; 2009.

12. Tillotson, AK, NH Tillotson, and R Abel. *The One Earth Herbal Sourcebook: Everything You Need to Know about Chinese, Western, and Ayurvedic Herbal Treatments.* New York, NY: Twin Streams; 2001.

Chamaemelum nobile and *Matricaria chamomilla:*

1. Tilgner, S. *Herbal Medicine: from the Heart of the Earth.* Pleasant Hill, OR: Wise Acres; 2009.

2. Hoffmann, D. *The New Holistic Herbal.* Shaftesbury, Dorset: Element; 1994.

3. Easley, T, and SH Horne. *The Modern Herbal Dispensatory: a Medicine-Making Guide.* Berkeley, CA: North Atlantic Books; 2016.

4. Balick, MJ, and A Weil. *Rodale's 21st-Century Herbal: a Practical Guide for Healthy Living Using Nature's Most Powerful Plants.* New York, NY: Rodale; 2014.

5. Nowell, H, E Birzneck, and DH College. *Chartered Herbalist Diploma Program.* Burnaby, BC, Canada: Dominion Herbal College; 2011.

6. Keefe, JR, JJ Mao, I Soeller, QS Li, and JD Amsterdam. "Short-term open label chamomile *(Matricaria chamomilla L.)* therapy of moderate to severe generalized anxiety disorder." *Phytomedicine.* 2016; 23(14): 1699-1705. Doi: 10.1016/j.phymed.2016.10.013.

7. Mao, JJ, SX Xie, JR Keefe, I Soeller, QS Li, and JD Amsterdam. "Long-term cham-omile *(Matricaria chamomilla L.)* treatment for generalized anxiety disorder: A randomized clinical trial." *Phytomedicine.* 2016; 23(14): 1735-1742. Doi: 10.1016/j. phymed.2016.10.012.

8. Amsterdam, JD, Y Li, I Soeller, K Rockwell, JJ Mao, and J Shults. "A Randomized, Dou-ble-Blind, Placebo-Controlled Trial of Oral *Matricaria recutita* (Chamomile) Extract Therapy for Generalized Anxiety Disorder." *Journal of Clinical Psychopharmacology.* 2009; 29(4): 378-382. Doi: 10.1097/ jcp.0b013e3181ac935c.

9. Taliou, A, E Zintzaras, L Lykouras, and K Francis. "An Open-Label Pilot Study of a Formulation Containing the Anti-Inflammatory Flavonoid Luteolin and Its Effects on Behavior in Children With Autism Spectrum Disorders." *Clinical Therapeutics.* 2013; 35(5): 592-602. Doi: 10.1016/ j.clinthera.2013.04.006.

10. Zargaran, A, A Borhani-Haghighi, M Salehi-Marzijarani, et al. "Evaluation of the effect of topical chamomile *(Matricaria chamomilla L.)* oleogel as pain relief in migraine without aura: a randomized, double-blind, placebo-controlled, crossover study." *Neurological Sciences.* 2018; 39(8): 1345-1353. Doi: 10.1007/s10072-018-3415-1.

11. Spinella, M. "Herbal Medicines and Epilepsy: The Potential for Benefit and Adverse Effects." *Epilepsy & Behavior.* 2001; 2(6): 524-532. Doi: 10.1006/ ebeh.2001.0281.

12. "German Chamomile Effectiveness, Safety, and Drug Interactions." *RxList.* https:// www.rxlist.com/german_chamomile/supplements.htm. Accessed January 15, 2019.

Cinnamomum verum and *Cinnamomum cassia:*

1. Pahan, K. "Prospects of Cinnamon in Multiple Sclerosis." *Journal of Multiple Scle-rosis.* 2015; 02(03). Doi: 10.4172/2376-0389.1000149.

2. Ho, S-C, K-S Chang, and P-W Chang. "Inhibition of neuroinflammation by cinnamon and its main components." *Food Chemistry.* 2013; 138(4): 2275-2282. Doi: 10.1016/j. foodchem.2012.12.020.

3. Maiolo, SA, P Fan, and L Bobrovskaya. "Bioactive constituents from cinnamon, hemp seed and polygonum cuspidatum protect against H_2O_2 but not rotenone toxicity in a cellular model of Parkinsons disease." *Journal of Traditional and Complementary Medicine.* 2018; 8(3): 420-427. Doi: 10.1016/j.jtcme.2017.11.001.

4. Momtaz, S, S Hassani, F Khan, M Ziaee, and M Abdollahi. "Cinnamon, a promising prospect towards Alzheimer's disease." *Pharmacological Research.* 2018; 130: 241-258. Doi: 10.1016/j.phrs.2017.12.011.

5. Peterson, DW, RC George, F Scaramozzino, et al. "Cinnamon Extract Inhibits Tau Aggregation Associated with Alzheimer's Disease In Vitro." *Journal of Alzheimer's Disease.* 2009; 17(3): 585-597. Doi: 10.3233/ jad-2009-1083.

6. Kannappan, R, SC Gupta, JH Kim, S Reuter, and BB Aggarwal. "Neuro-protection by Spice-Derived Nutraceuticals: You Are What You Eat!" *Molecular Neurobiology.* 2011; 44(2): 142-159. Doi: 10.1007/ s12035-011-8168-2.

7. Meamar, R, O Mirmosayyeb, A Tanhaei, et al. "Possible role of common spices as a preventive and therapeutic agent for Alzheimer's disease." *International Journal of Preventive Medicine.* 2017; 8(1): 5. Doi: 10.4103/ 2008-7802.199640.

Crocus sativus:

1. Lopresti, AL, and PD Drummond. "Saffron *(Crocus sativus)* for depression: a systematic review of clinical studies and examination of underlying antidepressant mechanisms of action." *Human Psychopharmacology: Clinical and Experimental.* 2014; 29(6): 517-527. Doi: 10.1002/hup.2434.

2. Moshiri, M, M Vahabzadeh, and H Hosseinzadeh. "Clinical Applications of Saffron *(Crocus sativus)* and its Constituents: A Review." *Drug Research.* 2014; 65(06): 287-295. Doi: 10.1055/s-0034-1375681.

3. Farokhnia, M, MS Sabet, N Iranpour, et al. "Comparing the efficacy and safety of *Crocus sativus L.* with memantine in patients with moderate to severe Alzheimer's disease: a double-blind randomized clinical trial." *Human Psychopharmacology: Clinical and Experimental.* 2014; 29(4): 351-359. Doi: 10.1002/hup.2412.

4. Finley, JW, and S Gao. "A Perspective on *Crocus sativus L.* (Saffron) Constituent Crocin: A Potent Water-Soluble Antioxidant and Potential Therapy for Alzheimer's Disease." *Journal of Agricultural and Food Chemistry.* 2017; 65(5): 1005-1020. Doi: 10.1021/acs.jafc.6b04398.

5. Akhondzadeh, S, MS Sabet, MH Harirchian, et al. "Saffron in the treatment of patients with mild to moderate Alzheimer's disease: a 16-week, randomized and placebo-controlled trial." *Journal of Clinical Pharmacy and Therapeutics.* 2010; 35(5): 581-588. Doi: 10.1111/j.1365-2710.2009.01133.x.

6. Moshiri, M, M Vahabzadeh, and H Hosseinzadeh. "Clinical Applications of Saffron *(Crocus sativus)* and its Constituents: A Review." *Drug Research.* 2014; 65(06): 287-295. Doi: 10.1055/s-0034-1375681.

7. Easley, T, and SH Horne. *The Modern Herbal Dispensatory: a Medicine-Making Guide.* Berkeley, CA: North Atlantic Books; 2016.

8. Balick, MJ, and A Weil. *Rodale's 21st-Century Herbal: a Practical Guide for Healthy Living Using Nature's Most Powerful Plants.* New York, NY: Rodale; 2014.

9. "Saffron Effectiveness, Safety, and Drug Interactions". *RxList.* https://www.rxlist. com/saffron/supplements.htm. Accessed January 15, 2019.

Cuminum cyminum:

1. Morshedi, D, F Aliakbari, A Tayaranian-Marvian, A Fassihi, F Pan-Montojo, and H Pérez-Sánchez. "Cuminaldehyde as the Major Component of *Cuminum cyminum,* a Natural Aldehyde with Inhibitory Effect on Alpha-Synuclein Fibrillation and Cytotoxicity." *Journal of Food Science.* 2015; 80(10). Doi: 10.1111/1750-3841.13016.

2. Wei, J, X Zhang, Y Bi, R Miao, Z Zhang, and H Su. "Anti-Inflammatory Effects of Cumin Essential Oil by Blocking JNK, ERK, and NF-κB Signaling Pathways in LPS-Stimulated RAW 264.7 Cells." *Evidence-Based Complementary and Alternative Medicine.* 2015; 2015: 1-8. Doi: 10.1155/2015/4745093.

3. "Cumin Effectiveness, Safety, and Drug Interactions." *RxList.* https://www.rxlist. com/cumin/supplements.htm#. Accessed December 22, 2018.

Curcuma longa:

1. Ringman, J, S Frautschy, G Cole, D Masterman, and J Cummings. "A Potential Role of the Curry Spice Curcumin in Alzheimer's Disease." *Current Alzheimer Research.* 2005; 2(2): 131-136. Doi: 10.2174/1567205053585882.

2. Ahmed, T, and A-H Gilani. "Therapeutic Potential of Turmeric in Alzheimer's Disease: Curcumin or Curcuminoids?" *Phytotherapy Research.* 2013; 28(4): 517-525. Doi: 10.1002/ptr.5030.

3. Chin, D, P Huebbe, K Pallauf, and G Rimbach. "Neuroprotective Properties of Curcumin in Alzheimer's Disease – Merits and Limitations." *Current Medicinal Chemistry.* 2013; 20(32): 3955-3985. Doi: 10.2174/09298673113209990210.

4. Goel, A, AB Kunnumakkara, and BB Aggarwal. "Curcumin as 'Curecumin': From kitchen to clinic." *Biochemical Pharmacology.* 2008; 75(4): 787-809. Doi: 10.1016/j. bcp.2007.08.016.

5. Gupta, SC, S Patchva, W Koh, and BB Aggarwal. "Discovery of curcumin, a component of golden spice, and its miraculous biological activities." *Clinical and Experimental Pharmacology and Physiology.* 2012; 39(3): 283-299. Doi: 10.1111/j.1440-1681.2011.05648.x.

6. Kim, DS, JY Kim, and Y Han. "Curcuminoids in Neurodegenerative Diseases." *Recent Patents on CNS Drug Discovery.* 2012; 7(3): 184-204. Doi: 10.2174/157488912803252032.

7. Mythri, RB, and MMS Bharath. "Curcumin: A Potential Neuroprotective Agent in Parkinson's Disease." *Current Pharmaceutical Design.* 2012; 18(1): 91-99. Doi: 10.2174/138161212798918995.

8. Ghanaatian, F, NA Lashgari, AH Abdolghaffari, et al. "Curcumin as a therapeutic candidate for multiple sclerosis: Molecular mechanisms and targets." *Journal of Cellular Physiology.* October 2018. Doi: 10.1002/ jcp.27965.

9. Bright, JJ. "Curcumin And Autoimmune Disease." *Advances In Experimental Medicine And Biology: The Molecular Targets and Therapeutic Uses of Curcumin in Health and Disease.* 2007: 425-451. Doi: 10.1007/978-0-387-46401-5_19.

10. Sun, J, F Chen, C Braun, et al. "Role of curcumin in the management of pathological pain." *Phytomedicine.* 2018; 48: 129-140. Doi: 10.1016/ j.phymed.2018.04.045

11. Kathrada, N, P Kory, T Lawrie, and P Mccullough. *Spike Protein Detox Guide.* 2023. Accessed August 14, 2023. https://worldcouncilforhealth.org/wpcontent/uploads/2023/03/SpikeProteinDetox_ENGLISH_V2FH.pdf

12. Greger, M, and G Stone. *How Not to Die: Discover the Foods Scientifically Proven to Prevent and Reverse Disease.* New York, New York: Flatiron Books; 2015.

13. Tilgner, S. *Herbal Medicine: from the Heart of the Earth.* Pleasant Hill, OR: Wise Acres; 2009.

14. Easley, T, SH Horne. *The Modern Herbal Dispensatory: a Medicine-Making Guide.* Berkeley, CA: North Atlantic Books; 2016.

15. Tillotson, AK, NH Tillotson, and R Abel. *The One Earth Herbal Sourcebook: Everything You Need to Know about Chinese, Western, and Ayurvedic Herbal Treatments.* New York, NY: Twin Streams; 2001.

16. Balick MJ, and A Weil. *Rodale's 21st-Century Herbal: a Practical Guide for Healthy Living Using Nature's Most Powerful Plants.* New York, NY: Rodale; 2014.

17. "Turmeric: Uses, Side Effects, Dosage, Interactions & Warning." *RxList.* https://www.rxlist.com/turmeric/supplements.htm. Accessed January 15, 2019.

Ginkgo biloba:

1. Wang, C, X Zhao, S Mao, Y Wang, X Cui, and Y Pu. "Management of SAH with traditional Chinese medicine in China." *Neurological Research.* 2006; 28(4) :436-444. Doi: 10.1179/016164106x115044.

2. Zhang, X, X-T Liu, and D-Y Kang. "Traditional Chinese Patent Medicine for Acute Ischemic Stroke." *Medicine.* 2016; 95(12). Doi: 10.1097/ md.0000000000002986.

3. D'Andrea, G, S Cevoli, and D Cologno. "Herbal therapy in migraine." *Neurological Sciences.* 2014; 35(S1): 135-140. Doi: 10.1007/ s10072-014-1757-x.

4. Bhidayasiri, R, O Jitkritsadakul, JH Friedman, and S Fahn. "Updating the recommendations for treatment of tardive syndromes: A systematic review of new evidence and practical treatment algorithm." *Journal of the Neurological Sciences.* 2018; 389: 67-75. Doi: 10.1016/j.jns.2018.02.010.

5. Chen, X, Y Hong, and P Zheng. "Efficacy and safety of extract of *Ginkgo biloba* as an adjunct therapy in chronic schizophrenia: A systematic review of randomized, double-blind, placebo-controlled studies with meta-analysis." *Psychiatry Research.* 2015; 228(1): 121-127. Doi: 10.1016/ j.psychres.2015.04.026.

6. Malik, J, S Choudhary, and P Kumar. "Plants and phytochemicals for Huntington's disease." *Pharmacognosy Reviews.* 2013; 7(14): 81-91. Doi: 10.4103/0973-7847.120505.

7. Niederhofer, H. "First preliminary results of an observation of *Ginkgo Biloba* treating patients with autistic disorder." *Phytotherapy Research.* 2009; 23(11): 1645-1646. Doi: 10.1002/ptr.2778.

8. Janssen, IM, S Sturtz, G Skipka, A Zentner, MV Garrido, and R Busse. "*Ginkgo biloba* in Alzheimer's disease: a systematic review." *Wiener Medizinische Wochenschrift.* 2010; 160(21-22): 539-546. Doi: 10.1007/ s10354-010-0844-8.

9. Oken, BS, DM Storzbach, and JA Kaye. "The Efficacy of *Ginkgo biloba* on Cognitive Function in Alzheimer's Disease." *Archives of Neurology.* 1998; 55(11): 1409-1415. Doi: 10.1001/archneur.55.11.1409.

10. Yang, G, Y Wang, J Sun, K Zhang, and J Liu. "*Ginkgo Biloba* for Mild Cognitive Impairment and Alzheimer's Disease: A Systematic Review and Meta-Analysis of Randomized Controlled Trials." *Current Topics in Medicinal Chemistry.* 2016; 16(5): 520-528. Doi: 10.2174/1568026615666150813143520.

11. Zhang, H-F, L-B Huang, Y-B Zhong, et al. "An Overview of Systematic Reviews of *Ginkgo biloba* Extracts for Mild Cognitive Impairment and Dementia." *Frontiers in Aging Neuroscience.* 2016; 8. Doi: 10.3389/ fnagi.2016.00276.

12. Spiegel, R, R Kalla, G Mantokoudis, et al. "*Ginkgo biloba* extract EGb 761® alleviates neurosensory symptoms in patients with dementia: a meta-analysis of treatment effects on tinnitus and dizziness in randomized, placebo-controlled trials." *Clinical Interventions in Aging.* 2018; Volume 13: 1121-1127. Doi: 10.2147/cia.s157877.

13. Easley, T, and SH Horne. *The Modern Herbal Dispensatory: a Medicine-Making Guide.* Berkeley, CA: North Atlantic Books; 2016.

14. Tilgner, S. *Herbal Medicine: from the Heart of the Earth.* Pleasant Hill, OR: Wise Acres; 2009.

15. Balick, MJ, and A Weil. *Rodale's 21st-Century Herbal: a Practical Guide for Healthy Living Using Nature's Most Powerful Plants.* New York, NY: Rodale; 2014.

16. Tillotson, AK, NH Tillotson, and R Abel. *The One Earth Herbal Sourcebook: Everything You Need to Know about Chinese, Western, and Ayurvedic Herbal Treatments.* New York, NY: Twin Streams; 2001.

17. Qiao, L, J Zheng, X Jin, et al. "Ginkgolic acid inhibits the invasiveness of colon cancer cells through AMPK activation." *Oncology Letters.* 2017; 14(5): 5831-5838. Doi: 10.3892/ol.2017.6967.

Hericium erinaceus:

1. Mori, K, S Inatomi, K Ouchi, Y Azumi, and T Tuchida. "Improving effects of the mushroom Yamabushitake *(Hericium erinaceus)* on mild cognitive impairment: a double-blind placebo-controlled clinical trial." *Phytotherapy Research.* 2009;23(3):367-372. Doi: 10.1002/ptr.2634.

2. Li, IC, LY Lee, TT Tzeng, et al. "Neurohealth Properties of *Hericium erinaceus* Mycelia Enriched with Erinacines." *Behav. Neurol.* 2018; 2018: 5802634. Published 2018 May 21. Doi: 10.1155/2018/5802634.

Hypericum perforatum:

1. Zirak, N, M Shafiee, G Soltani, M Mirzaei, and A Sahebkar. "*Hypericum perforatum* in the treatment of psychiatric and neurodegenerative disorders: Current evidence and potential mechanisms of action." *Journal of Cellular Physiology.* 2018. Doi: 10.1002/jcp.27781.

2. Ng, QX, N Venkatanarayanan, and CYX Ho. "Clinical use of *Hypericum perforatum* (St John's wort) in depression: A meta-analysis." *Journal of Affective Disorders.* 2017; 210: 211-221. Doi: 10.1016/j.jad.2016.12.048.

3. Apaydin, EA, AR Maher, R Shanman, et al. "A systematic review of St. John's wort for major depressive disorder." *Systematic Reviews.* 2016; 5(1). Doi: 10.1186/s13643-016-0325-2.

4. Galeotti, N. "*Hypericum perforatum* (St John's wort) beyond depression: A therapeutic perspective for pain conditions." *Journal of Ethnopharmacology.* 2017; 200: 136-146. Doi: 10.1016/j.jep.2017.02.016.

5. Rapkin, AJ, and EI Lewis. "Treatment of premenstrual dysphoric disorder." *Women's Health (London, England).* 2013; 9(6): 537-556. Doi: 10.2217/ whe.13.62.

6. Oliveira, AI, C Pinho, B Sarmento, and ACP Dias. "Neuroprotective Activity of *Hypericum perforatum* and Its Major Components." *Frontiers in Plant Science.* 2016; 7. Doi: 10.3389/fpls.2016.01004.

7. Easley, T, and SH Horne. *The Modern Herbal Dispensatory: a Medicine-Making Guide.* Berkeley, CA: North Atlantic Books; 2016.

8. Tilgner, S. *Herbal Medicine: from the Heart of the Earth.* Pleasant Hill, OR: Wise Acres; 2009.

9. Balick, MJ, and A Weil. *Rodale's 21st-Century Herbal: a Practical Guide for Healthy Living Using Nature's Most Powerful Plants.* New York, NY: Rodale; 2014.

10. Tillotson, AK, NH Tillotson, and R Abel. *The One Earth Herbal Sourcebook: Everything You Need to Know about Chinese, Western, and Ayurvedic Herbal Treatments.* New York, NY: Twin Streams; 2001.

11. Hoffmann, D. *The New Holistic Herbal.* Shaftesbury, Dorset: Element; 1994.

Nepeta cataria:

1. Tilgner, S. *Herbal Medicine: from the Heart of the Earth.* Pleasant Hill, OR: Wise Acres; 2009.

2. Hoffmann, D. *The New Holistic Herbal.* Shaftesbury, Dorset: Element; 1994.

3. Easley, T, and SH Horne. *The Modern Herbal Dispensatory: a Medicine-Making Guide.* Berkeley, CA: North Atlantic Books; 2016

4. Balick, MJ, and A Weil. *Rodale's 21st-Century Herbal: a Practical Guide for Healthy Living Using Nature's Most Powerful Plants.* New York, NY: Rodale; 2014.

5. Nowell, H, E Birzneck, and DH College. *Chartered Herbalist Diploma Program.* Burnaby, BC, Canada: Dominion Herbal College; 2011.

6. Gotter A. "Catnip Tea: Health Benefits and Uses." *Healthline.* Published November 15, 2017. Accessed October 12, 2023. https://www.health-line.com/health/catnip-tea.

Nigella sativa:

1. Forouzanfar, F, BS Bazzaz, and H Hosseinzadeh. "Black cumin *(Nigella sativa)* and its constituent (thymoquinone): a review on antimicrobial effects." *Iranian Journal of Basic Medical Sciences.* 2014; 17(12): 929-938.

2. Tavakkoli, A, A Ahmadi, BM Razavi, and H Hosseinzadeh. "Black Seed *(Nigella Sativa)* and its Constituent Thymoquinone as an Antidote or a Protective Agent Against Natural or Chemical Toxicities." *Iranian Journal of Pharmaceutical Research.* 2017; 16 (Suppl): 2-23.

3. Beheshti, F, M Khazaei, and M Hosseini. "Neuropharmacological effects of Nigella sativa." *Avicenna Journal of Phytomedicine.* 2016; 6(1): 104-116.

4. Jakaria, M, D-Y Cho, ME Haque, et al. "Neuropharmacological Potential and Delivery Prospects of Thymoquinone for Neurological Disorders." *Oxidative Medicine and Cellular Longevity.* 2018; 2018: 1-17. Doi: 10.1155/ 2018/1209801.

5. Kathrada, N, P Kory, T Lawrie, and P Mccullough. *Spike Protein Detox Guide.* 2023. Accessed August 14, 2023. https://worldcouncilforhealth.org/wp-content/uploads/2023/03/SpikeProteinDetox_ENGLISH_V2FH.pdf.

6. Ahmad, A, A Husain, M Mujeeb, et al. "A review on therapeutic potential of *Nigella sativa:* A miracle herb." *Asian Pacific Journal of Tropical Biomedicine.* 2013; 3(5): 337-352. Doi: 10.1016/s2221-1691(13)60075-1.

7. Hosseinzadeh, H, A Tavakkoli, V Mahdian, and BM Razavi. "Review on Clinical Trials of Black Seed *(Nigella sativa)* and Its Active Constituent, Thymoquinone." *Journal of Pharmacopuncture.* 2017; 20(3): 179-193. Doi: 10.3831/kpi.2017.20.021.

8. Dajani, EZ, TG Shahwan, and NE Dajani. "Overview of the Preclinical Pharmacological Properties of *Nigella Sativa* (Black Seeds): A Complementary Drug with Historical and Clinical Significance." *Journal of Physiology and Pharmacology.* 2016; 67(6): 801-817.

9. "Black Seed Effectiveness, Safety, and Drug Interactions". *RxList.* https://www.rxlist.com/ black_seed/supplements.htm. Accessed January 1, 2019.

Passiflora spp.:

1. Ozarowski, M, PŁ Mikołajczak, and B Thiem. "[Medicinal plants in the phytotherapy of alcohol or nicotine addiction. Implication for plants in vitro cultures]". *Przeglad Lekarski.* 2013; 70(10): 869-874.

2. Kargozar, R, H Azizi, and R Salari. "A review of effective herbal medicines in controlling menopausal symptoms." *Electronic Physician.* 2017; 9(11): 5826-5833. Doi: 10.19082/5826.

3. Mani, R, and V Natesan. "Chrysin: Sources, beneficial pharmacological activities, and molecular mechanism of action." *Phytochemistry.* 2018; 145: 187-196. Doi: 10.1016/j.phytochem.2017.09.016.

4. Miroddi, M, G Calapai, M Navarra, P Minciullo, and S Gangemi. *"Passiflora incarnata L.*: Ethnopharmacology, clinical application, safety and evaluation of clinical trials." *Journal of Ethnopharmacology.* 2013; 150(3): 791-804. Doi: 10.1016/j.jep.2013.09.047.

5. Sarris, J. "Herbal medicines in the treatment of psychiatric disorders: 10-year updated review." *Phytotherapy Research.* 2018; 32(7): 1147-1162. Doi: 10.1002/ptr.6055.

6. Krenn, L. "[Passion Flower *(Passiflora incarnata L.)*—a reliable herbal sedative]." *Wiener Medizinische Wochenschrift* (1946). 2002; 152(15-16): 404-406.

7. Wheatley, D. "Medicinal plants for insomnia: a review of their pharmacology, efficacy and tolerability." *Journal of Psychopharmacology* (Oxford, England). 2005; 19(4): 414-421.

8. Hoffmann, D. *The New Holistic Herbal.* Shaftesbury, Dorset: Element; 1994.

9. Easley, T, and SH Horne. *The Modern Herbal Dispensatory: a Medicine-Making Guide.* Berkeley, CA: North Atlantic Books; 2016.

10. Tilgner, S. *Herbal Medicine: from the Heart of the Earth.* Pleasant Hill, OR: Wise Acres; 2009.

11. Balick, MJ, and A Weil. *Rodale's 21st-Century Herbal: a Practical Guide for Healthy Living Using Nature's Most Powerful Plants.* New York, NY: Rodale; 2014.

12. Cunha, JP. "Passion Flower: Side Effects, Dosages, Treatment, Interactions, Warnings." *RxList.* https://www.rxlist.com/consumer_passion_flower/drugs-condition.htm. Accessed January 2, 2019.

Phyllanthus emblica:

1. Baliga, MS, and JJ Dsouza. "Amla *(Emblica officinalis Gaertn)*, a wonder berry in the treatment and prevention of cancer." *European Journal of Cancer Prevention.* 2011; 20(3): 225-239. Doi: 10.1097/cej.0b013e32834473f4.

2. Yadav, SS, MK Singh, PK Singh, and V Kumar. "Traditional knowledge to clinical trials: A review on therapeutic actions of *Emblica officinalis*." *Biomedicine & Pharmacotherapy.* 2017; 93: 1292-1302. Doi: 10.1016/j.biopha.2017.07.065.

3. Tillotson, AK, NH Tillotson, and R Abel. *The One Earth Herbal Sourcebook: Everything You Need to Know about Chinese, Western, and Ayurvedic Herbal Treatments.* New York, NY: Twin Streams; 2001.

4. "Indian Gooseberry Effectiveness, Safety, and Drug Interactions." *RxList.* https://www.rxlist.com/indian_gooseberry/supplements.htm. Accessed January 2, 2019.

Piper methysticum:

1. Gounder, R. "Kava consumption and its health effects." *Pacific Health Dialog.* 2006; 13(2): 131-135.

2. Sarris, J, E Laporte, and I Schweitzer. "Kava: A Comprehensive Review of Efficacy, Safety, and Psychopharmacology." *Australian & New Zealand Journal of Psychiatry.* 2011; 45(1): 27-35. Doi: 10.3109/00048674.2010.522554.

3. Smith, K, and C Leiras. "The effectiveness and safety of Kava Kava for treating anxiety symptoms: A systematic review and analysis of randomized clinical trials." *Complementary Therapies in Clinical Practice.* 2018; 33: 107-117. Doi: 10.1016/j. ctcp.2018.09.003.

4. Tillotson, AK, NH Tillotson, and R Abel. *The One Earth Herbal Sourcebook: Everything You Need to Know about Chinese, Western, and Ayurvedic Herbal Treatments.* New York, NY: Twin Streams; 2001.

5. Tilgner, S. *Herbal Medicine: from the Heart of the Earth.* Pleasant Hill, OR: Wise Acres; 2009.

6. Easley, T, and SH Horne. *The Modern Herbal Dispensatory: a Medicine-Making Guide.* Berkeley, CA: North Atlantic Books; 2016.

7. Balick, MJ, and A Weil. *Rodale's 21st-Century Herbal: a Practical Guide for Healthy Living Using Nature's Most Powerful Plants.* New York, NY: Rodale; 2014.

8. "Kava Effectiveness, Safety, and Drug Interactions." *RxList.* https://www.rxlist.com/ kava/supplements.htm. Accessed January 5, 2019.

9. Murray, MT, and JE Pizzorno. *The Encyclopedia of Natural Medicine.* 3rd ed. New York, NY: Atria Paperback (Simon & Schuster); 2012.

Punica granatum:

1. Asgary, S, S Javanmard, and A Zarfeshany. "Potent health effects of pomegranate." *Advanced Biomedical Research.* 2014; 3(1): 100. Doi: 10.4103/ 2277-9175.129371.

2. Jurenka, J. "Therapeutic Applications of Pomegranate (Punica granatum L.): A Review." *Alternative Medicine Review.* 2008; 13(2): 128-144.

3. Nowell, H, E Birzneck, and DH College. *Chartered Herbalist Diploma Program.* Burnaby, BC, Canada: Dominion Herbal College; 2011.

4. Hoffmann, D. *The New Holistic Herbal.* Shaftesbury, Dorset: Element; 1994.

5. Balick, MJ, and A Weil. *Rodale's 21st-Century Herbal: a Practical Guide for Healthy*

Living Using Nature's Most Powerful Plants. New York, NY: Rodale; 2014.

6. "Pomegranate Effectiveness, Safety, and Drug Interactions." *RxList.* https://www.rxlist.com/pomegranate/supplements.htm. Accessed January 6, 2019.

Rosmarinus officinalis:

1. de Oliveira, MR. "The Dietary Components Carnosic Acid and Carnosol as Neuroprotective Agents: a Mechanistic View." *Molecular Neurobiology.* 2015; 53(9): 6155-6168. Doi: 10.1007/s12035-015-9519-1.

2. Habtemariam, S. "The Therapeutic Potential of Rosemary *(Rosmarinus officinalis)* Diterpenes for Alzheimer's Disease." *Evidence-Based Complementary and Alternative Medicine.* 2016; 2016: 1-14. Doi: 10.1155/2016/2680409.

3. Ayaz, M, A Sadiq, M Junaid, F Ullah, F Subhan, and J Ahmed. "Neuro-protective and Anti-Aging Potentials of Essential Oils from Aromatic and Medicinal Plants." *Frontiers in Aging Neuroscience.* 2017; 9. Doi: 10.3389/ fnagi.2017.00168.

4. Tilgner, S. *Herbal Medicine: from the Heart of the Earth.* Pleasant Hill, OR: Wise Acres; 2009.

5. Hoffmann, D. *The New Holistic Herbal.* Shaftesbury, Dorset: Element; 1994.

6. Easley, T, and SH Horne. *The Modern Herbal Dispensatory: a Medicine-Making Guide.* Berkeley, CA: North Atlantic Books; 2016.

7. Balick, MJ, and A Weil. *Rodale's 21st-Century Herbal: a Practical Guide for Healthy Living Using Nature's Most Powerful Plants.* New York, NY: Rodale; 2014.

8. Cunha, JP. "Rosemary: Side Effects, Dosages, Treatment, Interactions, Warnings." *RxList.* https://www.rxlist.com/consumer_rosemary/drugscondition.htm. Accessed January 6, 2019.

9. "Rosemary Effectiveness, Safety, and Drug Interactions." *RxList.* https://www.rxlist.com/rosemary/supplements.htm. Accessed January 6, 2019.

Scutellaria baicalensis/Scutellaria lateriflora:

1. Gasiorowski, K, E Lamer-Zarawska, J Leszek, et al. "Flavones from Root of *Scutellaria Baicalensis Georgi:* Drugs of the Future in Neurodegeneration?" *CNS & Neurological Disorders -Drug Targets.* 2011; 10(2): 184-191. Doi: 10.2174/187152711794480384.

2. Ashbaugh, A, and C Mcgrew. "The Role of Nutritional Supplements in Sports Concussion Treatment." *Current Sports Medicine Reports.* 2016; 15(1): 16-19. Doi: 10.1249/jsr.0000000000000219.

3. Liang, W, X Huang, and W Chen. "The Effects of Baicalin and Baicalein on Cerebral Ischemia: A Review." *Aging and Disease.* 2017; 8(6): 850-867. Doi: 10.14336/ad.2017.0829.

4. Sowndhararajan, K, P Deepa, M Kim, S Park, and S Kim. "Neuroprotective and Cognitive Enhancement Potentials of Baicalin: A Review." *Brain Sciences.* 2018; 8(6): 104. Doi: 10.3390/brainsci8060104.

5. Tillotson AK, NH Tillotson, and R Abel. *The One Earth Herbal Sourcebook: Everything You Need to Know about Chinese, Western, and Ayurvedic Herbal Treatments.* New York, NY: Twin Streams; 2001.

6. "Baikal Skullcap Effectiveness, Safety, and Drug Interactions." *RxList.* https://www.rxlist.com/baikal_skullcap/supplements.htm. Accessed January 7, 2019.

7. Setzer, WN. "The Phytochemistry of Cherokee Aromatic Medicinal Plants." *Medicines (Basel, Switzerland).* 2018; 5(4): 121. Doi: 10.3390/medicines5040121.

8. Tilgner, S. *Herbal Medicine: from the Heart of the Earth.* Pleasant Hill, OR: Wise Acres; 2009.

9. Hoffmann, D. *The New Holistic Herbal.* Shaftesbury, Dorset: Element; 1994.

10. Easley, T, and SH Horne. *The Modern Herbal Dispensatory: a Medicine-Making Guide.* Berkeley, CA: North Atlantic Books; 2016.

11. Nowell, H, E Birzneck, and DH College. *Chartered Herbalist Diploma Program.* Burnaby, BC, Canada: Dominion Herbal College; 2011.

12. "Skullcap Effectiveness, Safety, and Drug Interactions." *RxList.* https://www.rxlist.com/skullcap/supplements.htm. Accessed January 7, 2019.

Syzygium aromaticum:

1. Fujisawa, S, and Y Murakami. "Eugenol and Its Role in Chronic Diseases." *Advances in Experimental Medicine and Biology Drug Discovery from Mother Nature.* 2016: 45-66. Doi: 10.1007/978-3-319-41342-6_3.

2. Liu, Q, X Meng, Y Li, C-N Zhao, G-Y Tang, and H-B Li. "Antibacterial and Antifungal Activities of Spices." *International Journal of Molecular Sciences.* 2017; 18(6): 1283. Doi: 10.3390/ijms18061283.

3. Tsuchiya, H. "Anesthetic Agents of Plant Origin: A Review of Phytochemicals with Anesthetic Activity." *Molecules*. 2017; 22(8): 1369. Doi: 10.3390/ molecules22081369.

4. Cortés-Rojas, DF, CRFD Souza, and WP Oliveira. "Clove *(Syzygium aromaticum)*: a precious spice." *Asian Pacific Journal of Tropical Biomedicine*. 2014; 4(2): 90-96. Doi: 10.1016/s2221-1691(14)60215-x.

5. "Clove Effectiveness, Safety, and Drug Interactions." *RxList*. https://www.rxlist. com/clove/ supplements.htm. Accessed January 7, 2019.

6. Hoffmann, D. *The New Holistic Herbal*. Shaftesbury, Dorset: Element; 1994.

7. Balick, MJ, and A Weil. *Rodale's 21st-Century Herbal: a Practical Guide for Healthy Living Using Nature's Most Powerful Plants*. New York, NY: Rodale; 2014.

8. Nowell, H, E Birzneck, and DH College. *Chartered Herbalist Diploma Program*. Burnaby, BC, Canada: Dominion Herbal College; 2011.

9. Easley, T, and SH Horne. *The Modern Herbal Dispensatory: a Medicine-Making Guide*. Berkeley, CA: North Atlantic Books; 2016.

Vaccinium myrtillus:

1. Smeriglio, A, D Monteleone, and D Trombetta. "Health Effects of *Vaccinium myrtillus L.*: Evaluation of Efficacy and Technological Strategies for Preservation of Active Ingredients." *Mini-Reviews in Medicinal Chemistry*. 2014; 14(7): 567-584. Doi: 10.2174/1389557514666140722083034.

2. Cunha, JP. "Bilberry: Side Effects, Dosages, Treatment, Interactions, Warnings." *RxList*. https://www.rxlist.com/consumer_bilberry/drugscondition.htm. Accessed January 8, 2019.

3. "Bilberry Effectiveness, Safety, and Drug Interactions." *RxList*. https://www.rxlist. com/bilberry/supplements.htm. Accessed January 8, 2019.

4. Easley, T, and SH Horne. *The Modern Herbal Dispensatory: a Medicine-Making Guide*. Berkeley, CA: North Atlantic Books; 2016.

5. Balick, MJ, and A Weil. *Rodale's 21st-Century Herbal: a Practical Guide for Healthy Living Using Nature's Most Powerful Plants*. New York, NY: Rodale; 2014.

6. Tillotson AK, NH Tillotson, and R Abel. *The One Earth Herbal Sourcebook: Everything You Need to Know about Chinese, Western, and Ayurvedic Herbal Treatments*. New York, NY: Twin Streams; 2001.

7. Tilgner, S. *Herbal Medicine: from the Heart of the Earth*. Pleasant Hill, OR: Wise Acres; 2009.

8. "Blueberry Effectiveness, Safety, and Drug Interactions." *RxList.* https://www.rxlist.com/blueberry/supplements.htm. Accessed January 8, 2019.

Valeriana officinalis:

1. Hadley, S, and JJ Petry. "Valerian." *American Family Physician.* 2003; 67(8): 1755-1758.

2. Anheyer, D, R Lauche, D Schumann, G Dobos, and H Cramer. "Herbal medicines in children with attention deficit hyperactivity disorder (ADHD): A systematic review." *Complementary Therapies in Medicine.* 2017; 30: 14-23. Doi: 10.1016/j.ctim.2016.11.004.

3. Mojaverrostami, S, MN Bojnordi, M Ghasemi-Kasman, MA Ebrahimzadeh, and HG Hamidabadi. "A Review of Herbal Therapy in Multiple Sclerosis." *Adv Pharm Bull.* 2018; 8(4): 575-590.

4. Ghazanfarpour, M, R Sadeghi, S Abdolahian, and RL Roudsari. "The efficacy of Iranian herbal medicines in alleviating hot flashes: A systematic review." *International Journal of Reproductive BioMedicine (Yazd, Iran).* 2016; 14(3): 155-166. Doi: 10.29252/ijrm.14.3.155.

5. Maleki-Saghooni, N, FZ Karimi, Z Behboodi Moghadam, and K Mirzaii Najmabadi. "The effectiveness and safety of Iranian herbal medicines for treatment of premenstrual syndrome: A systematic review." *Avicenna J Phytomed.* 2018; 8(2): 96-113.

6. "Valerian Effectiveness, Safety, and Drug Interactions." *RxList.* https://www.rxlist.com/valerian/supplements.htm. Accessed January 8, 2019.

7. Cunha, JP. "Valerian: Side Effects, Dosages, Treatment, Interactions, Warnings." *RxList.* https://www.rxlist.com/consumer_valerian/drugscondition.htm. Accessed January 8, 2019.

8. Tilgner, S. *Herbal Medicine: from the Heart of the Earth.* Pleasant Hill, OR: Wise Acres; 2009.

9. Hoffmann, D. *The New Holistic Herbal.* Shaftesbury, Dorset: Element; 1994.

10. Easley, T, and SH Horne. *The Modern Herbal Dispensatory: a Medicine-Making Guide.* Berkeley, CA: North Atlantic Books; 2016.

11. Balick, MJ, and A Weil. *Rodale's 21st-Century Herbal: a Practical Guide for Healthy Living Using Nature's Most Powerful Plants.* New York, NY: Rodale; 2014.

12. Nowell, H, E Birzneck, and DH College. *Chartered Herbalist Diploma Program.* Burnaby, BC, Canada: Dominion Herbal College; 2011.

13. Tillotson AK, NH Tillotson, and R Abel. *The One Earth Herbal Sourcebook: Everything You Need to Know about Chinese, Western, and Ayurvedic Herbal Treatments.* New York, NY: Twin Streams; 2001.

Zingiber officinale:

1. Mojaverrostami, S, MN Bojnordi, M Ghasemi-Kasman, MA Ebrahimzadeh, and HG Hamidabadi. "A Review of Herbal Therapy in Multiple Sclerosis." *Adv Pharm Bull.* 2018; 8(4): 575-590.

2. Jafarzadeh, A, and M Nemati. "Therapeutic potentials of ginger for treatment of Multiple sclerosis: A review with emphasis on its immunomodulatory, anti-inflammatory and anti-oxidative properties." *Journal of Neuroimmunology.* 2018; 324: 54-75. Doi: 10.1016/j.jneuroim.2018.09.003.

3. Aggarwal, BB, and S Shishodia. "Suppression of the Nuclear Factor-κB Activation Pathway by Spice-Derived Phytochemicals: Reasoning for Seasoning." *Annals of the New York Academy of Sciences.* 2004; 1030(1): 434-441. Doi: 10.1196/annals.1329.054.

4. Rahmani, AH, FM Shabrmi, and SM Aly. "Active ingredients of ginger as potential candidates in the prevention and treatment of diseases via modulation of biological activities." *Int J Physiol Pathophysiol Pharmacol.* 2014; 6(2): 125-36. Published 2014 Jul 12.

5. Choi, JG, SY Kim, M Jeong, and MS Oh. "Pharmacotherapeutic potential of ginger and its compounds in age-related neurological disorders." *Pharmacology & Therapeutics.* 2018; 182: 56-69. Doi: 10.1016/ j.pharmthera.2017.08.010.

6. Tilgner, S. *Herbal Medicine: from the Heart of the Earth.* Pleasant Hill, OR: Wise Acres; 2009.

7. Hoffmann, D. *The New Holistic Herbal.* Shaftesbury, Dorset: Element; 1994.

8. Easley, T, and SH Horne. *The Modern Herbal Dispensatory: a Medicine-Making Guide.* Berkeley, CA: North Atlantic Books; 2016.

9. Balick, MJ, and A Weil. *Rodale's 21st-Century Herbal: a Practical Guide for Healthy Living Using Nature's Most Powerful Plants.* New York, NY: Rodale; 2014.

10. Nowell, H, E Birzneck, and DH College. *Chartered Herbalist Diploma Program.* Burnaby, BC, Canada: Dominion Herbal College; 2011.

11. Tillotson, AK, NH Tillotson, and R Abel. The One Earth Herbal Sourcebook: Everything You Need to Know about Chinese, Western, and Ayurvedic Herbal Treatments.

New York, NY: Twin Streams; 2001.

12. "Ginger Effectiveness, Safety, and Drug Interactions." *RxList.* https://www.rxlist.com/ginger/supplements.htm. Accessed January 9, 2019.

13. Cunha, JP. "Ginger (African Ginger): Side Effects, Dosages, Treatment, Interactions, Warnings." *RxList.* https://www.rxlist.com/consumer_ginger_african_ginger/drugs-condition.htm. Accessed January 9, 2019.

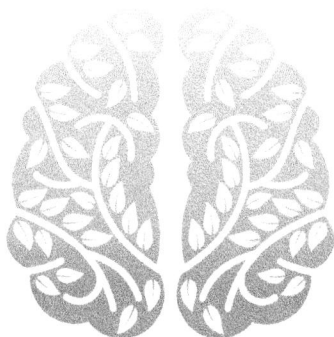

CHAPTER 2

Important Issues

Big Picture Healing

It is important to understand the big-picture view of how healing occurs. Whether this is new information or a review, it is worth taking the time for an overview. While I have seen this model in different forms, in this review I want to utilize Dr. Dietrich Klinghardt's model as a basis for the discussion.[1] It should be noted that Naturopathic Medicine's view of healing is similar to this model. In any case, Dr. Klinghardt's model envisions five levels related to health. Work on the lower levels provides energy and the basis for work on the higher levels. Treatments that affect the higher levels can filter down to create healing on the lower levels. In general, it is important to address all five levels of healing.

The first level is the physical level (which includes things such as nutrition, herbs, environmental medicine and toxicology, osteopathic and structural medicine, etc.). The second level is the energetic level and includes work such as acupuncture and the impact of electromagnetic fields on health. The third level is profoundly tied to psychology and issues such as trauma. The fourth level includes topics such as family and trans-generational issues, among others. The fifth level is the spiritual level, which can include the idea of God/Goddess, religion, spirituality, ethics, meaning, and purpose in life. Prayer and finding deep meaning in one's work and life belong in this realm. I find this model to be very useful in guiding healing and providing a framework for organizing the various treatment approaches. It certainly applies to neurological and psychological disorders, as well as to health-related issues in general.

Confusion, Diagnostic and Therapeutic Issues, and the Complexity of Healing Options

I want to note that there are serious concerns about the effect of misdiagnosis on patients. Without a proper diagnosis, treatments may fail to work. The differential diagnosis process is crucial to guiding healing. In the conventional medical world, sometimes attempts are made to cut costs and save time during the diagnostic process. This can lead to misdiagnosis which can be devastating for patients in terms of the possibility of healing.

The differential diagnostic process should be thorough. Physical and organic causes of disease should be found. Conventional medicine can be fantastic in this process when the healthcare provider is not trying to cut corners. All potential causative factors in neuropsychiatric symptoms should be clarified. Laboratory work, physical examination, diagnostic imaging (with preference being given to techniques such as MRI, thermography, and ultrasound whenever safely possible to avoid ionizing radiation), and history-taking are invaluable.

In addition to the conventional diagnostic process, and while certainly not a replacement, I believe there may be tremendous value in utilizing other methods of obtaining diagnostic knowledge. I've seen various techniques over the years, including muscle testing, bioresonance testing, and energy-medicine-based diagnoses. I recommend caution when approaching these methods. Their value may be based on the skill of the practitioner, and I think relying on them exclusively as a guide for treatment can be dangerous under specific circumstances. You may miss an important diagnosis or the method may generate inaccurate results and lead you down a wrong path. Still, they can be useful in the hands of a skilled practitioner as a supplement to conventional diagnostic processes. I particularly like medical intuition. As in any field, there are practitioners of medical intuition who have high accuracy and those who do not. Dr. Cay Randall-May is an example of an outstanding medical intuitive.[1] The National Organization for Medical Intuition (NOMI) is a resource in this field.[2] A talented medical intuitive can really make a positive difference in guiding treatment. If, however, one depends only on a medical intuitive who has low accuracy, without using any conventional diagnostic information, the outcome may be disastrous.

It is very important not to fall into the belief that anything alternative is good and anything conventional is bad. There are dangerous practices and ways of thinking in both conventional and alternative medicine. Use common sense and intuition along with research to guide yourself. Yes, nature should be a guide, but there are things in alternative medicine that are not natural. Having a rigid belief system that rejects anything conventional can leave you susceptible to incorrect and dangerous methods of treatment and unethical practitioners. Some practitioners may be well-meaning but susceptible to their own bias against conventional medicine. Gentle natural treatments can be wonderfully beneficial. Harsh unnatural treatments that are labeled as "alternative" can be promoted simply because they are outside of conventional medicine, and this can be extraordinarily dangerous. Sometimes a natural substance may not work, and studies should not be automatically dismissed because they show something natural lacks efficacy. The substance may not have efficacy, and the study may be valid. On the other hand, studies may be biased, and funding sources and potential bias should be looked into. The point is to not always automatically determine whether a treatment is efficacious or not based on whether it is conventional or alternative, but instead to carefully consider each treatment with an open mind.

Therapeutic options in alternative medicine can be overwhelming in their sheer numbers. There is a seemingly endless supply of systems and modes of therapy to try, in the hope that something will work. This can, as one can imagine, cost a significant amount in terms of both financial resources and time. And while one of these options may prove effective, the person may grow increasingly desperate if nothing seems to be working. The overall goal of this work is to somewhat simplify the massive amount of information out there into some kind of framework to facilitate healing. Please keep in mind that healing does not always have to be expensive and cost-prohibitive. Sometimes the simplest treatments may be effective. Doing more is not always better. Sometimes doing less is actually more effective in terms of treatment options.

It is possible to go down a path of alternative medicine which is profoundly costly and may not provide a positive outcome. Finding the cause of the problem should help lead to the simplest and most cost-effective solution. Focus on the basics. It is possible to be told by well-meaning practitioners that you feel worse because of a healing crisis. This is certainly possible, but if this healing crisis persists, it is very important to evaluate whether the treatment is making things worse. My feeling is that healing crises should be short. In general, if one is on the right path, they will feel better. A healing crisis may not occur at all. You may simply feel better. There may be ups and downs, but patients should feel that they are on the right path in general. These are simple ideas that can be useful in general, but obviously do not apply to every situation.

I want to add some notes about the issue of chronic Lyme disease. Please be careful with chronic Lyme disease treatment which involves long-term antibiotic therapy. I am not saying that this mode of treatment is never beneficial to patients—it may benefit some patients. But there are a lot of problems in the current treatment of Lyme disease. From the conventional side, I think the idea that Lyme disease cannot be a chronic infection is faulty. It does seem to sometimes become chronic Lyme disease. But from the other side of the debate, the solution of long-term antibiotic treatment can be devastating in terms of side effects. An untreated Lyme disease infection certainly can also be devastating. I speak with a great deal of personal experience on this issue. There are some people who may have more serious issues to treat, and even though they have Lyme disease, it may not be the primary cause of their health problems. To focus on this specific infection while ignoring other issues can put the patient through a tremendous amount of suffering, in addition to being financially problematic. In the end, they may see no benefit after all of that effort. Lyme disease is an important issue. It should not be ignored. Mold is an important issue. It should not be ignored. There are many potential causes of neurological symptoms that should not be ignored. There are too many patients who are being treated for only one issue, and this approach may or may not benefit them. Always keep a big picture view of things. If you only focus on one issue, you may get better, but you could also lose a significant amount of time and resources without any benefit. This can cause a loss of hope in patients.

Ironically, some alternative medicine practitioners tend to be the most supportive of long-term antibiotic therapy for Lyme disease. Just be careful with this approach. Don't damage your body with long-term antibiotic therapy, which has questionable efficacy, without really thinking it through. I actually agree with the more conventional view of not treating Lyme disease with long-term antibiotics. People may remain sick for many reasons, including inflammation, autoimmunity, nutrition, etc. They may still have an active infection, but long-term treatment of that is better done through natural and gentle methods. The immune system should be optimized, and the many recommendations related to lifestyle (nutrition, sleep, EMFs, social support, etc.) discussed in this book should be followed. Herbal medicine can be utilized to address chronic Lyme disease. Homeopathy can also be utilized in this regard.

Traditional Chinese medicine and Ayurvedic medicine are also big-picture styles of healing that can be useful with numerous chronic diseases. Talented homeopathic practitioners can be extraordinary healers and really facilitate improvement in health. Do not underestimate the healing power of homeopathy, whether classical, complex, or nosode/causative styles. When there are multiple diagnoses and confusion, a skilled healthcare provider can guide the patient by treating the core issues. Sometimes secondary diagnostic findings will go away without specific treatment. Having a talented healthcare provider working with you is necessary in complex cases.

Environmental Medicine

Environmental medicine must be considered in any plan to address neurological conditions. Minimizing exposure to all potential toxins should be a priority. This includes avoiding neurotoxins. Eating a 100%

organic diet and using 100% organic products in the home and on the body minimizes exposure to harmful synthetic pesticides, insecticides, and herbicides. Eating a 100% plant-based diet (supplemented with vitamin B12) dramatically lowers toxin exposure. For example, dioxin exposure can be lowered by approximately 95% by eliminating animal products from the diet.[1] This occurs because of the effects of bio-magnification (with toxin concentration increasing higher on the food chain). Maximize raw, steamed, or boiled food intake and avoid high-temperature cooking (such as baking and frying). This will minimize the intake of acrylamide, a neurotoxin.[2]

Drinking and showering in filtered water helps minimize toxins. Avoid water in plastic bottles, which is an environmental catastrophe. In some places, the tap water is of such high quality (e.g., the Netherlands) that a home water filtration system may not be necessary.[3] Otherwise, the use of home water filtration may be appropriate.

Minimize exposure to plastics as much as possible throughout daily life. This includes items which come into contact with food and drink. Avoid plastic bottles, plastic wraps, plastic containers, etc. Plastics in general should also be avoided, whether they are food-related or not, for environmental and health purposes.

Heavy metals exposure should be minimized. In particular, mercury, aluminum, and lead should be avoided. Mercury may be present in batteries, fluorescent light bulbs, mercury amalgam dental fillings, old thermometers, seafood, areas near coal power plants, and in some vaccines.

Aluminum exposure may occur through aluminum-treated drinking water, antiperspirants, baking powder, aluminum cookware, aluminum foil, some vaccines, and dialysis. Whenever possible, avoid drugs that list aluminum as an ingredient.

Lead exposure can occur from old paint, batteries, leaded gasoline, and lead-containing water pipes. In children, lead exposure is linked to lowered intelligence and behavioral and attention-related issues.[4] Fetal mercury exposure negatively affects brain development.

Alzheimer's disease may be associated with lead, mercury, arsenic, cadmium, and aluminum exposure.[5] Parkinson's disease may be linked to exposure to lead, pesticides, and solvents.

In general, preventing exposure is the best method. If exposure to toxins has already occurred, stop any further exposure. The body continually attempts to detoxify itself, with varying degrees of success. Water-only fasting is very beneficial in accelerating this process (see the section on fasting later in this chapter for precautions and details). Garlic should be considered as a treatment for lead poisoning.[6] Refer to the section on *Allium sativum* (Garlic) for further details related to this plant.

Electromagnetic fields (EMFs) are a significant public health issue and must be considered when discussing environmental medicine. Electromagnetic field exposure occurs through electricity, power lines, electrical devices, cell phones, microwave ovens, wireless internet, wireless routers, wireless devices, smart meters, radars, etc. EMF exposure may be associated with breast cancer, allergies/ inflammation, miscarriage, neurodegenerative diseases, leukemia, genotoxicity, and brain tumors.[7] Maximum effort must be made to minimize exposure to electromagnetic fields, for both general and neurological health. Minimize the use of technology in general, particularly in the bedroom and when sleeping. Use wired technology instead of wireless. Landlines are preferred over cellphones. Wired internet should be chosen over wireless; utilize wired routers in place of wireless routers. This issue must be addressed aggressively to ensure optimal neurological well-being. Children's Health Defense, founded by Robert F. Kennedy Jr., does very important work in bringing to light how environmental issues, including EMFs, may negatively impact health.[8]

I want to thank Dr. Savely Yurkovsky[9] for bringing to my attention the negative impact of EMFs on treatment outcomes and efficacy. Continued EMF exposure can prevent healing and impede the efficacy of other treatments.

Please minimize and preferably eliminate your exposure to tobacco smoke and alcohol. Refer to the sections on Addiction and Trauma Healing in Chapter 3 for help with addictive behaviors.

As a final note, please pay attention to the inactive ingredients in supplements. Sometimes these ingredients have potential negative health impacts over the long term. This may be theoretical, but it is always better to avoid unnecessary ingredients. For example, whenever possible, I recommend avoiding things like magnesium stearate (a lubricant). Supplements should be as clean and simple as possible in terms of both active and inactive ingredients.

Exercise

Physical activity is well-known as a vital component of health. It would also be expected to be important as part of neurological disease prevention and treatment. Indeed, the scientific literature seems to support that notion. In Parkinson's disease, aerobic exercise appears to be beneficial in terms of slowing the disease's progress.[1] In fact, all forms of physical activity appear to be beneficial in Parkinson's disease treatment, including resistance training, traditional Chinese exercise, yoga, and dancing.[2] In Alzheimer's disease treatment, exercise may provide significant benefits with respect to quality of life, general health, and neurological and psychiatric outcomes.[3] In multiple sclerosis, exercise should be included as a component of a successful treatment program, providing significant benefits to patients, including improving their quality of life, functional capacity, and cognitive function.[4-5] The utilization of exercise in Huntington's disease may lead to beneficial results, including with respect to gait speed, motor function, and balance.[6]

A remarkably thorough review of the scientific literature concluded that there is evidence supporting the prevention of a minimum of 35 medical conditions through exercise and that exercise is effective in the treatment of 26 conditions, including schizophrenia, anxiety, depression, multiple sclerosis, Parkinson's disease, coronary heart disease, cancer, and dementia.[7] Interestingly, exercise appears to be helpful in the prevention of both Alzheimer's disease and vascular dementia. The evidence is clear. Exercise must be incorporated into any wellness program for both prevention and treatment of neurological conditions. Patients should check with their physician to ensure that they can engage in an exercise program safely, particularly if they have any underlying medical conditions. There are an incredible variety of activities which involve physical activity. Each person should consult with their physician as part of determining the best form of exercise for them. What is appropriate will differ from person to person, depending on overall health, specific disease conditions, etc. This process will help determine the ideal type of exercise or combination of exercises for each situation. Most important is to find something that the person enjoys doing and can participate in safely. As a general guideline for general health and for prevention of diseases, at least 90 minutes per day of moderate exercise is recommended.[8]

Fasting

Fasting has varied definitions. There is dry fasting, which is the exclusion of all substances (food and water). Water-only fasting allows water and excludes all other substances. Juice fasting allows fresh vegetable juice, fresh fruit juice, and water but excludes all other substances. There are many variations of fasting, including time-restricted eating (for example only eating during an eight-hour window of the day and not eating for the other sixteen hours). Some people fast 1 day per week and others undergo monthly, seasonal, or yearly fasts. Fasting has the potential to aid in the prevention and treatment of Huntington's disease, Parkinson's disease, and Alzheimer's disease.[1] There is also potential for benefiting patients with neurological damage (such as from stroke or traumatic brain injury). Caution is necessary with respect to fasting in cases of amyotrophic lateral sclerosis, and it may be contraindicated. Fasting can promote autophagy and DNA repair (even with short fasts of 16 hours to 48 hours). Fasting for longer than 48 hours increases stem-cell regeneration.

While it is not an exaggeration to state that fasting is remarkable and must be considered one of the primary effective methods of treatment and prevention for nearly all human diseases, the benefits, side effects, contraindications, precautions, and other issues must be addressed in more detail.[2-8] Fasting is the body's method of healing. When something is wrong, the body in many cases shuts down appetite, encouraging the energy of digestion to be focused on healing whatever issue is of concern. In the process of fasting, damaged body parts are broken down, fat is utilized for energy, toxins are removed from the body, and massive amounts of energy are focused on healing any and all damaged tissue in the body. The body, in a sense, is renewed and regenerated during the

fasting period and in the post-fast period of rebuilding. As stated earlier, this process involves stem-cell regeneration. The incredibly broad
variety of mechanisms of action associated with fasting gives it the
potential to address nearly all neurological conditions. This includes the
potential to directly repair or confront the underlying causative factors
involved in these conditions. If the neurological condition is caused by
heavy metal toxicity or other toxin exposure, fasting addresses this. If
the condition is caused by neurological damage, fasting may potentially
address this through the removal of damaged cells or cell components
and stem-cell regeneration. If there is an issue of leaky gut syndrome or
other digestive issues causing neurological conditions, fasting can help
address this. In neurological conditions associated with atherosclerosis,
fasting may help dissolve the plaques. If a neurological condition is
associated with autoimmunity, fasting may function to reset the entire
immune system, reducing autoimmunity and thereby improving the
condition. In fact, it is difficult to think of an area in neurology where
fasting could not be potentially useful (with the possible exception of
amyotrophic lateral sclerosis). Fasting should be considered part of a
healthy lifestyle for virtually all people, for both general health and
wellness and for neurological concerns. Fasting also has use in psychiatry (which can be thought of as intimately connected to neurology),
boasting a 70% effectiveness rate in chronic schizophrenia.[9]

Of course, there are contraindications and concerns related to therapeutic fasting. Generally, most authorities on fasting recommend that
fasting not be utilized by pregnant women and people under the age of
18. Fasting should generally not be utilized in people with eating disorders unless they are under strict medical supervision. People whose
body mass index (BMI) is very low should not fast. Those on medications
require medical supervision, particularly with medications affecting

blood glucose and blood pressure, anti-depressants, anti-convulsants, and corticosteroids. In general, fasting authorities recommend avoiding fasting for people with Type-1 diabetes. Rarely, people can lack the genetic ability to successfully adapt to ketosis, and they obviously should not fast.

In people with gallstones, caution and medical supervision are absolutely necessary. It would seem wise to adopt a plant-based diet along with specific herbal therapy directed toward gall bladder issues for a period of time before undergoing fasting, in order to reduce the likelihood of complications during the fasting process.

For generally healthy individuals with no medical conditions who do not take any medications, water-only fasting is very safe for up to 3 days. If the water-only fast is longer than 5 days, medical supervision is always required, even in healthy individuals. Minor conditions can benefit from shorter fasts. However, serious conditions sometimes require a water fast lasting between 14 and 40 days. For general health and maintenance, there are various recommendations: longer fasts would be less frequently done, for example, once a year or less, while shorter fasts could be done seasonally, monthly, or weekly. From all of the evidence and recommendations, however, it would seem logical to fast for at least 3 days in order to gain some of the deeper levels of healing that occur in the post-48-hour period.

Medical supervision is always beneficial with fasting, because people can experience very distressing symptoms during the process prior to achieving remarkable results. Nausea and vomiting are common. They are generally not serious when occurring in the earlier part of the fast but can be very serious if occurring toward the end of the fast. Diarrhea can occur. Headaches, skin rashes, body odor, fatigue, weakness, and many other possible symptoms may appear or worsen during the fast. Fainting can occur and should be guarded against. Patients should stand slowly, avoid hot showers, move their legs if they are sitting or standing for extended periods of time, and they should lay down if they feel they are going to faint. Medical guidance is helpful to differentiate between serious symptoms and the so-called "healing crisis" symptoms. The fasting process can be extraordinarily challenging, but with perseverance, dramatic outcomes can occur, changing people's lives. Temporary discomfort from these symptoms is generally followed by improved health. Most authorities recommend ending the fast if the person has healed the condition or conditions of concern, if the person simply cannot psychologically continue, if a serious heart rhythm abnormality is being observed, if severe weakness is present, or if vomiting is severe. In addition, electrolytes should be checked weekly during the fast, as abnormal potassium levels would suggest it is time to end the fast. A return of strong hunger is also an indicator that it is time to end the fast. Body temperature, weight/ BMI, pulse, and blood pressure should probably be checked twice a day for any fast longer than 3 days and definitely for any fast longer than 5 days.

Breaking the fast must be done carefully. This point cannot be emphasized enough. Severe digestive disturbances can result from breaking the fast too quickly with too much food. A small amount of food, the size of the patient's fist, can be taken every two hours to break the fast. This amount can slowly increase, as tolerated over a period of time equaling half of the fasting length. For example, if the fast was 14 days, the amount of food would be slowly increased over 7 days to normal quantities. Fruits and vegetables are good at the beginning of breaking a fast. Other plant foods like whole grains, nuts, and seeds can be added after 3-4 days of breaking the fast. Beans should be added last.

Following these guidelines helps in minimizing the risk of "re-feeding syndrome" and the digestive problems that can occur post-fasting. In conclusion, water-only fasting should be a fundamental component of neurology, as it enhances the possibility of maximizing health. It should be combined with a plant-based diet (in between the water fasts) and appropriate herbs for the prevention and treatment of nearly all neurological conditions.

While this section introduces this topic, it is not meant to be an exhaustive review of all the issues involved with water-only fasting. Physicians experienced in supervising water-only fasting should be involved in patient care as part of the healing team in all cases where the fast lasts more than 5 days.

Gastrointestinal Health

There is a significant connection between the digestive system and neurological and psychological health. The general health recommendations throughout this work are likely to benefit the gastrointestinal system. It should be noted that stress and trauma can negatively impact the digestive system.[1] In particular cases, where the digestion requires some added attention, Dr. Zach Bush has been involved in creating a product that supports the health of the gastrointestinal system.[2] In specific cases with significant digestive system involvement in the neurological or psychological symptoms, the use of this digestive support product may be very beneficial.

Important Considerations for Finding Supportive Healthcare Providers

It is important for people to have supportive healthcare providers in their lives. Whether a physician, herbalist, nutritionist, massage therapist, psychologist, or any other provider, the choice of healthcare provider is vital. While knowledge and types of treatment offered are important, I have found through experience that a practitioner's bedside manner is crucial. Unfortunately, in healthcare, as in all fields, there are practitioners who may lack compassion and empathy. They may be overly critical or too dogmatic. Sometimes they are authoritarian in their style. While some people may respond positively to various personality styles, I think it is important for the patient to feel safe, supported, and heard. The patient should feel that the person cares about them and that their time is not rushed. If you feel like a healthcare provider is dismissive, if they lack compassion and empathy, or if you don't feel safe around them, please change healthcare providers. If you have a feeling that the healthcare provider is viewing you simply as a means of extracting money, please find another practitioner. People for whom finances are the priority do exist in the healthcare field, and they can be very detrimental to the patient. While everyone needs to make a living, there should be clear empathy, compassion, and motivation to heal coming from the practitioner. Trust your intuition. Please keep in mind that healthcare providers can, like any human, have toxic personalities, which may be abusive. These healthcare providers should be avoided if at all possible. If something feels wrong, there's a decent chance it is wrong. In patients with psychological symptoms such as paranoia, it can be difficult to reality-test. Please share your concerns about the healthcare provider with someone you trust and try to make

decisions based on objective reality as best you can. We need more compassion, empathy, and kindness in healthcare and less profit motive.
Finding positive practitioners to support your path toward health is
profoundly important.

Infectious Agents

Neurological function can be profoundly affected by infectious agents,
including viral, bacterial, fungal, and parasitic infections. Infectious
agents have been linked to multiple sclerosis, amyotrophic lateral sclerosis, and Alzheimer's disease.[1] For example, Alzheimer's disease may be
tied to Human Herpes Virus 1, Human Herpes Virus 2, Cytomegalovirus,
Hepatitis C, *Treponema denticola*, and *Porphyromonas gingivalis.*[2] Epstein-
Barr virus is linked to multiple sclerosis.[3] Parkinson's disease may be
tied to *Helicobacter pylori.*[4] Schizophrenia is associated with *Toxoplasma
gondii.*[5] Lyme disease (*Borrelia burgdorferi*) may be associated with a
wide range of neuropsychiatric issues, including obsessive-compulsive
disorder, anorexia nervosa, bipolar disorder, depression, panic attacks,
schizophrenia, dementia, autism, seizures, and Alzheimer's disease.[6] As a
side note, it should be noted that cinnamon, cloves, and garlic may have
significant potential for the treatment of Lyme disease.[7-8] Conventional
medicine may have lifesaving applications in terms of infectious disease
treatment depending on the infection and specific circumstances, and it
is beyond the scope of this work to discuss conventional pharmaceutical
treatment of infectious diseases. Only a patient, in consultation with
their healthcare provider, can decide when conventional pharmaceutical medications should be utilized.

However, the overall issue here is to note that infections have a
significant role in neurology. When selecting herbs for consideration in

herbal neurology, antiviral, antibacterial, anti-fungal, and anti-parasitic properties may be very useful. The plants discussed in the first chapter of this book include many useful herbs against infectious agents. Plants with potential antiviral effects include: *Allium sativum*, *Curcuma longa*, *Hypericum perforatum*, *Nigella sativa*, *Passiflora spp.*, *Phyllanthus emblica*, *Syzygium aromaticum*, and *Zingiber officinale*. Plants with potential antibacterial effects include: *Allium sativum*, *Curcuma longa*, *Hypericum perforatum*, *Nigella sativa*, *Phyllanthus emblica*, *Syzygium aromaticum*, and *Zingiber officinale*. Antifungal properties are associated with: *Allium sativum*, *Curcuma longa*, *Hypericum perforatum*, *Nigella sativa*, *Phyllanthus emblica*, *Syzygium aromaticum*, and *Zingiber officinale*. Anti-parasitic properties are associated with: *Allium sativum*, *Curcuma longa*, *Nigella sativa*, *Punica granatum*, and *Syzygium aromaticum*. Refer to each plant entry individually (in Chapter 1) for details, precautions, contraindications, and dosages. It should also be noted that putting too much attention on the infection and not enough on the entire patient would appear to be a mistake.

Strengthening the overall health of the individual increases resistance to all infections and should be the priority. Finally, water-only fasting (see the entry on fasting above for details) has strong potential to be a broad therapy for infectious agents, along with other causative factors associated with neurological conditions (autoimmunity, heavy metals, neurotoxins, atherosclerosis, inflammation).

Inner Work

While the area of inner work may seem vague, it is fundamental to living a meaningful and healthy life. In our childhood, sometimes, we are exposed to difficult events or styles of parenting that can create long-lasting negative effects. It is very important, for example, to learn to guide our lives based on love, compassion, and empathy, instead of being driven by anxiety, guilt, and shame.[1] Dr. Peter Breggin's work is fundamental to understanding these issues. To be driven by guilt does not generally make someone a more ethical human being. Doing things for positive reasons (love) is much healthier and more sustainable. This issue requires some deep introspection but can have very meaningful effects on our lives. For example, being driven by guilt can set someone up for a lifetime of abusive and toxic relationships. It can make people vulnerable to mistreatment. As a result, not dealing with these issues increases the likelihood of negative neurological and psychological consequences of stress, which can include PTSD. It is stressful to be abused in relationships, and the brain is sensitive to stress. Doing this inner work helps to create resistance to abusive relationships in our lives and gives more meaning to our daily living.

Along those same lines, it can be helpful to remove negative contracts we have with ourselves.[2] Sarah Peyton's work may be very helpful in this regard. These contracts with ourselves can stem from childhood and open us up to a lifetime of abuse and self-sabotage. Becoming aware of these negative contracts with ourselves and releasing them may be a useful form of inner work. It may increase our resistance to toxic relationships. Since toxic relationships can have negative effects on our neurological and psychological health, increasing resistance to them and reducing the likelihood of getting into one of these relationships is very beneficial.

The work of Dr. Joe Dispenza is also very valuable in terms of inner work. It is my belief that Dr. Dispenza's work may help with the manifestation of positive outcomes in life, increasing the likelihood of positive relationships, reducing the likelihood of toxic relationships, improving overall and neurological and psychological health, and allowing us to live a more meaningful life. Dr. Dispenza's work may also increase compassion, empathy, love, and abundance in life (which can minimize economic stress). There are two meditations related to love and inspiration which I highly recommend.[3-4] Oprah Winfrey's work also can be extremely helpful in supporting inner work and healing.[5-6] In addition, Anita Moorjani's writing is inspirational in guiding us toward authenticity.[7]

I want to also discuss working on our inner programming, which is formed in early childhood. These inner beliefs have a profound influence on our lives. Dr. Bruce H. Lipton discusses this issue, and his work is very useful when doing inner work.[8] A technique which may be very useful in changing this childhood programming (when it is problematic due to adverse childhood experiences) is PSYCH-K®.[9] I do think this technique can help with addressing negative beliefs and transforming them into positive ones. As a component of a more comprehensive inner work program, it can be very helpful. I have doubts that it is sufficient in and of itself as a system for addressing very complex cases. But it is a useful tool to keep in mind when doing inner work.

Mind-Body Medicine

Mind-body medicine should be incorporated into any overall wellness plan.[1-2] It should also be a part of any program to address neurological conditions. Stress management is vital. Meditation, yoga, and breathing exercises can be useful. Exercise may serve as a form of stress management.

Having a strong support system and loving relationships is important. Maximize your social support by connecting with family and friends (and forming new friendships and relationships if your social support is currently inadequate). You can read more about this in the section entitled "Relationships and Health," below. Healing past trauma promotes good health. (Also see the section on post-traumatic stress disorder in Chapter 3.) Psychologists can help people heal from such traumas. Various techniques can be utilized for releasing trauma, including EMDR (Eye Movement Desensitization and Reprocessing), the letter writing technique, etc.

Psychoanalysis and cognitive-behavioral therapy may improve quality of life. Living an ethical life is important. Positive thinking should also be a part of mind-body medicine and can make a significant difference in a person's quality of life. Fulfilling one's purpose in life would also seem to be important for achieving overall health. Finally, prayer and spirituality may have beneficial effects on health. In summary, addressing issues within the realm of mind-body medicine should have a positive impact on both overall and neurological health.

Nutrition

Proper nutrition is a must for everyone, including those dealing with neurological diseases. I recommend that people consume a whole-food vegan diet for optimal neurological and overall health, based on overwhelming scientific evidence.[1-8] This recommended diet contains no animal products (no meat, fish, dairy, or eggs) and no processed foods (nothing with refined grains, added sugar, added salt, or added oil). The ideal diet contains whole grains, beans, fruits, vegetables, nuts, seeds, and mushrooms and should be supplemented with vitamin B12. Vitamin B12 is produced by bacteria, and due to modern sanitation, everyone needs a vitamin B12 supplement. Individual food sensitivities should be addressed within the context of this diet. Consuming raw, sprouted, steamed, or boiled foods within this diet further improves the diet by avoiding toxins formed by cooking at high temperatures (acrylamide and advanced glycation end products).[9-10]

An organic whole-food vegan diet free of added salt/oil/sugar should be utilized as a component of an overall plan to prevent and treat Parkinson's disease.[8,11-13] Organic plant foods should be maximized, because of the relationship between pesticides and Parkinson's disease. Toxins and pesticides must be minimized, and this is done by eliminating animal products (which concentrate toxins, chemicals, and pesticides through bio-magnification) and by exclusively eating ecologically-cultivated, organic plant foods. Dairy products are particularly guilty in association with Parkinson's disease. Foods that may be particularly beneficial with respect to Parkinson's disease include berries and bell peppers. Tomatoes, eggplant, and potatoes may also be helpful. Supplementation with vitamin B12 is necessary.

The same organic, whole-food, vegan diet, free of added salt/ oil/ sugar should also be utilized for the prevention and treatment of multiple sclerosis.[14-15] While the evidence from a controlled trial was a bit disappointing, it did demonstrate the possibility of improving fatigue in MS patients through the consumption of the diet described above. This trial was short-term and cannot be relied upon for understanding the long-term effects of this diet. The work of Dr. Roy Swank appears to be more meaningful, showing remarkably positive results over decades of monitoring the use of a low-fat diet in multiple sclerosis patients. Dr. Swank seemed to believe that animal-based saturated fats were highly involved in the development of multiple sclerosis. To address not only multiple sclerosis but also overall health, it would be wise to adopt an organic, wholefood, vegan diet low in saturated fat. This diet should be free of added salt/oil/sugar. In addition, as a precaution, coconut and cacao should be strictly limited to minimize saturated fat. Nuts, seeds, and avocado should not be consumed in excess. In fact, in the case of multiple sclerosis, other than ground chia seeds, hemp seeds, or flax seeds for essential fatty acids, fatty plant foods should be avoided. While it may be that plant-based saturated fat does not worsen multiple sclerosis (Dr. Swank put emphasis on animal-based saturated fat contributing to multiple sclerosis), these steps are done out of an abundance of caution. Again, it is important to supplement with vitamin B12.

The brain is dependent on a healthy vascular system. A diet to prevent and treat neurological disorders must be a diet that is beneficial for the vascular system. An organic, whole-food, vegan diet with zero added sugar, zero added oil, and zero added salt should maximize the likelihood of preventing and reversing vascular disease.[1,4,5,8,16-22] In fact, there is compelling scientific evidence suggesting that this type of diet may help in the prevention of essentially all the common causes of death in the United States.[8] Thus, this dietary advice applies to essentially everyone. Along with supplemental vitamin B12, this diet is the foundation for the prevention and treatment of neurological disease. It should be standard care for herbalists to discuss nutrition with their patients. And this type of dietary advice complements herbal medicine nicely. After all, the scientific evidence demonstrates that we should be maximizing our intake of whole plants (and mushrooms). Maximizing whole plant foods maximizes the positive contributions to health inherent in these foods.

And eliminating animal products eliminates exposure to negative substances such as heme iron, cholesterol, animal-based protein, animal-based fat, and prions. Herbalists are interested in the effects of plants on human beings. Plants should be our medicine, through our diet and by complementing that diet with additional herbal medicine when necessary.

The organic, whole-food, vegan diet supplemented with vitamin B12 is the ideal diet for the prevention and treatment of neurological diseases, and for general health optimization. In addition, it has profound ethical benefits. According to the World Watch Institute, up to 51% of global greenhouse gas emissions are from livestock.[23] The United Nations estimate is lower, at 18%. However, regardless, following this diet is an ethical imperative to save the planet from climate change. The environmental consequences of animal agriculture are devastating. Another ethical benefit derived from following this diet relates to the animals themselves. Worldwide, approximately 70 billion animals are slaughtered annually in the animal agriculture industry.[24] This number is so ethically shocking that it calls for dramatic action. Adopting the organic, whole-food, vegan diet improves human health, addresses climate change, and improves the well-being of animals. Considerations of diet cannot only be concerned with human health but must account for the entirety of the consequences of choices people make. This recommended diet addresses these issues in the most positive manner possible.

There is the possibility of extremely rare genetic conditions that may require external supplementation of things like carnitine.[25] For nearly everyone else, the general recommendations above are advised. Nearly 100% of the population is covered by these general recommendations. If someone has an extremely rare genetic condition requiring animal-based nutrients, please seek supplementation with a vegan-sourced supplement, if at all possible. This maximizes the health of the individual with the genetic condition while also maximizing the ethics under those circumstances. Obviously, if a vegan-sourced supplement is not available, one can solve the rare genetic health issue with non-vegan supplements or food, but that is less preferable if there is a vegan-sourced alternative.

I want to add a personal note on the issue of salt in the diet. This issue is a bit controversial, and from my perspective, many people can tolerate a bit of salt. It may also be that some people do better with a small amount of added salt. Again, in general, I think the above recommendations (100% plant-based, no-salt/no-sugar/no-oil added, B12 supplemented, iodine sufficient) are ideal for most people. Please do include some sea vegetables for sufficient iodine (recommended intake of sea vegetables varies by type due to varying iodine content). Having general blood testing done regularly is recommended, as it can help optimize various issues that may arise, such as vitamin D, iron, and vitamin B12 levels. Women may need to address iron deficiency issues and men may need to address zinc deficiency. And within the plant-based diet, some people do better with less fat (fewer nuts, seeds, avocado, coconut) and others may do better with more whole plant-food-based fats (more nuts, seeds, avocado, coconut). I believe if healthy weight loss is a desired goal, in general one can go with a lower-fat, whole-food, plant-based diet. People will have to explore the various amounts of nuts/ seeds/avocado/coconut that they do best on. The default recommendation should be not too much fat, but everyone is different.

There is significant anatomical and physiological evidence demonstrating that humans are herbivores.[26] For the details demonstrating that humans are herbivores, please refer to the work of Dr. Milton Mills. Culturally, historically, and out of necessity under specific circumstances, humans can adapt to omnivorous diets, but that does not make it the ideal diet for health. Of course, there are genetic variations that may create differences in how well someone may tolerate animal products. In extremely rare genetic cases, as mentioned above, animal products or supplementation with vegan-created supplements (example: carnitine) may be necessary. But these are the extraordinarily rare exceptions, not the general rule. Please keep the anatomic evidence of humans being herbivores in mind as a general rule when planning your diet. There can also be cases of "withdrawal"-type symptoms when people switch to a plant-based diet. This is not a reason to go back to the unhealthy diet. These symptoms should resolve with time, as the body adapts to the diet it was designed for. If it does not, that may require further investigation into whether specific supplementation may be necessary (example: carnitine). Please see the work of Dr. Michael Klaper for more information on this withdrawal issue.[27-29]

The issue of essential fatty acids is a bit controversial. There are different schools of thought. On one end of the spectrum, it is believed that you don't need to think about essential fatty acids on a plant-based diet as long as added oils are restricted. Others talk about adding some walnuts, hemp seeds, ground flax seeds, or ground chia seeds to ensure optimum intake. At the other end of the spectrum are people who recommend adding vegan EPA/ DHA supplementation. I personally think that avoiding added oils combined with including a small amount of walnuts, hemp seeds, ground flax seeds, or ground chia seeds in the diet should be sufficient in general. If someone wants to add the vegan EPA/DHA supplement for insurance (or fears about the fatty acid conversion process being insufficient), I think that's reasonable too. The people who don't think about essential fatty acids at all as long as added oils are restricted probably will do fine as well, but everyone's different, and maybe we should be flexible about where everyone lands on this spectrum. I tend to be more cautious, so I would lean toward addressing the essential fatty acid issue through one or both of the options above (instead of ignoring it). In any case, it is my hope that the complex issue of nutrition has been simplified a bit, and the importance of nutrition has become evident in terms of neurological and overall health.

Raising Children

The method by which we raise children is vital to supporting their healthy psychological and neurological development. It is beyond the scope of this work to go into significant details regarding childrearing practices, but the work of Gabor Maté and Gordon Neufeld is highly recommended.[1-2] Children should be, to the maximum extent possible, raised in loving, compassionate environments, with many caring adults involved in their upbringing (a village or tribal or community set-up). Punitive methods of raising children are discouraged. Time-out and crying-it-out methods are discouraged. The child should never feel that the attachment relationship to the parent is dependent on their behavior. Rather, boundaries can be set in as gentle a manner as possible, while maintaining the unconditional love that provides secure attachment. That basic attachment should never be threatened in response to challenging behavior. Gentle guidance, boundary setting, and modeling positive behavior can help guide development while forming secure attachments. This can help children find their authentic selves while feeling secure in their attachment to their caregivers.

There are many issues related to pregnancy, pre-conception, conception, and childbirth which also can have long-term effects on the psychological and neurological development of children. Minimizing stress levels should be a societal goal, not just an individual task.

Economic stress, violence, and discrimination can have negative impacts on neuropsychological development. Improving nutrition can also provide significant benefits during childhood. The environment always matters and is certainly important while the brain is developing. To the maximum extent possible, and consistent with safety on an individually-determined basis, attempting to replicate our developmental patterns from our long historical evolution will likely yield positive results. There are profound benefits to breastfeeding and natural childbirth. Certainly, it is not always possible to breastfeed, and the birthing process can require medical intervention in a small percentage of cases to ensure the safety of mother and child, but in general, it is good to encourage breastfeeding and natural childbirth, but without guilt or shame if the individual decides for whatever reason to take a different path. Every individual must decide what is right for them based on personal preference and safety.

Please avoid or at least minimize trauma to children as much as possible. For example, during childbirth, avoid cutting the umbilical cord until it stops pulsating. This has huge benefits for the child. Cutting the cord too early can be very harmful psychologically. Dr. Michel Odent discusses the importance of these types of considerations.

In addition, both male and female circumcision should be eliminated, unless medically necessary or chosen by the person themselves when they reach the age of consent. This will help reduce trauma. I am aware that there are strong religious, cultural, and tradition-based beliefs involved in circumcision. We must respect religious, cultural, and traditional beliefs to the maximum extent possible. However, when these beliefs conflict with fundamental human rights, human rights must take priority. Here, as in the past, these beliefs can be adapted to meet human rights standards. I speak here as someone who was subjected to traditional male circumcision as an infant. It is an act that violates the integrity of the infant's body and is done without the child's consent. It is not reversible and is not acceptable, regardless of religious, cultural, or tradition-based justifications. We should support keeping the positive aspects and interpretations of religions, cultures, and traditions while leaving behind those aspects which violate human rights.

Relationships and Health

The impact of relationships on our neurological and psychological health is profound. We need healthy relationships to survive and thrive. Loneliness also has a deeply negative impact on our health.[1] We need positive, healthy relationships, and simultaneously must avoid unhealthy relationships. Understanding the difference between healthy and unhealthy relationships requires significant education because it is not commonly understood. Everyone should spend some time studying the basics of toxic relationships, including the issue of narcissism. Dr. Ramani Durvasula's work is profoundly useful in this education process.[2-4] Avoiding or removing yourself from abusive relationships, whether romantic, with a family member, or at the workplace, is an important goal. Sometimes complete avoidance or removal from the situation is not possible or the person simply does not prefer this route, and in this case, particular strategies can be employed to minimize the damage of maintaining these relationships. High-conflict, antagonistic, toxic people have a negative impact on the health of those around them. This form of stress negatively impacts the brain. One can certainly develop PTSD from a toxic relationship. The issue of personality disorders and toxic behaviors actually has a broader impact worldwide with respect to health than many people realize. The work of Dr. Noam Chomsky, Dr. Ramani Durvasula, Dr. Jordan Peterson, and Dr. Phil McGraw help shed light on this important phenomenon.

Publicly-traded corporations on Wall Street actually require/ encourage behavior that can sometimes be antisocial (resembling the behavior of a sociopath/psychopath). Placing profits above any moral, ethical, health, and environmental issues has a negative impact on neurological health and health in general. It also moves us toward the possibility of human extinction in terms of the climate change crisis. In addition, people with personalities that tend to lack conscientious- ness tend to accumulate in positions of power (heads of corporations, politicians, extraordinarily wealthy billionaires, famous celebrities). Of course, this is not to indict everyone who is part of these groups, but there tends to be a higher proportion of people with problematic personalities in these groups.

Anti-social personality disorder and narcissistic personality disorders are highly problematic and create severe issues on the individual level and on a societal level in terms of health and well-being, especially when these people are in positions of power. For the survival of the human species, these issues must become common knowledge. Everyone needs to be educated on these issues in order to protect ourselves from such dangerous people. People who consistently lack empathy should not be granted extraordinary power to control people's lives and make decisions on behalf of others. Another recommendation is to be wary of communal narcissists, who appear to be very caring people on the outside but can be quite dangerous underneath their superficial kindness. Protecting ourselves does not mean lacking compassion for others. We can have compassion and empathy for these dangerous people while simultane- ously protecting ourselves with boundaries, knowledge, and avoidance.

I did want to add some important points related to boundaries and removing or limiting psychologically toxic people from your life. Depending on the nature of your relationship with the psychologically toxic person (partner, spouse, parent, child, friend, co-worker, boss, etc.), you will need to decide how to proceed in terms of minimizing the harm from these relationships. Every situation is different, and each person must make their own decisions. If at all possible, eliminating contact completely is generally the best solution. If that is not possible, limiting contact as much as possible may be helpful. Sometimes, limiting conversations to nonemotional (boring) topics can minimize harm. It is important to understand that sometimes these types of people search for conflict or create conflict out of nothing or something small in order to provoke a reaction from you. You must learn and understand all the vocabulary associated with personality disorders, including the traits of narcissism. This person's behavior may get worse if you do not allow yourself to be provoked (although hopefully only temporarily), but eventually, the hope is that the person will get bored and move on. Vocabulary terms such as baiting, narcissistic supply, no contact, tension reduction, etc., need to be studied in order to protect yourself. Again Dr. Ramani Durvasula's work is profoundly important in this regard.

I do recommend always having the contact information of a good lawyer, because you may need one when dealing with high-conflict people. Do not hesitate to call on law enforcement if there are threats to your safety. And qualified therapists are vital in helping one move through such difficult situations—but the therapist must be knowledgeable about narcissism. Learning martial arts/self-defense may also prove useful if you need to defend yourself against violence. For defending yourself as peacefully as possible, Aikido is particularly recommended.

Even if you do not ever need to defend yourself physically, learning martial arts improves self-confidence and increases the feeling of safety.

In dangerous living situations, it can also be beneficial to have an emergency bag packed and ready to go. This should include important documents (ID, passport, birth certificate, for example), cash, vital or difficult-to-replace items, and perhaps some clothes. Basically, this is a bag you can grab in an emergency to leave easily and quickly. Obviously, the dangerous person in your life should not know about this bag. Be aware of your surroundings and have a plan on how to exit a situation whenever you know you are entering a situation/place with someone who has toxic personality traits. Obviously, these things exist on a spectrum, and some of these preparations may not be applicable or necessary. But it is good to be prepared for potentially dangerous situations if you are spending time with someone exhibiting dangerous personality traits.

Please familiarize yourself with the idea of trauma bonding, which is a form of addiction to the person abusing you. It is not the victim's fault that they feel addicted to someone who is not healthy for them. This relates to childhood wounds in the victim, typically similarities between caregivers from childhood and the abusive partner. It also can reflect the biochemistry of the roller coaster ups and downs of conflict in these types of relationships. It can be extraordinarily difficult to leave abusive relationships. Have compassion for yourself or anyone who is essentially attempting to break an addiction. This is not a place for judgment or criticism. One of the most helpful tips from Dr. Ramani Durvasula is making as complete a record as possible of all the negative things that the abuser has done to you. Reviewing this list can help prevent relapse into the abusive relationship. There is no substitute for making this list. While some people may be able to break free of the addiction without it, the chances of success probably increase by putting in the time to make the list. Please keep in mind the idea of euphoric recall—that is, our memories can paint a more positive reflection of the events of the relationship (minimizing how bad it really was). As with any addiction, if relapse occurs, be gentle with yourself. You can try again to leave the abusive relationship if you want and learn from the relapse. Keep in mind that the abuser will likely use your relapse to make you feel guilty, thereby attempting to keep you stuck in the relationship. Their manipulative tactics can make it more difficult to leave the relationship with every relapse, as the guilt increases. Do not allow guilt and manipulation to control your decision-making. Get as much healthy social support as possible after a break-up and take time to find yourself. Get in touch with the core of your being and take care of your health as much as possible. It is extremely important to do psychological self-work in order to prevent future toxic relationships. It takes work to change the patterns of being attracted to someone who is not healthy for you. Doing this work will increase the chances of having healthier relationships in the future.

Sometimes the feeling of being separated from the abuser in your life can feel like the end of the world. This feeling is very real to anyone breaking out of any addiction, including a trauma bond. The feeling will pass, but you need healthy distractions to get you through this time. Focus on things that are important to you—hobbies, meaningful work, volunteering, healthy social support (friends, family). Sometimes, you can feel better for a while, and then all of a sudden you will miss the person. This feeling can be very strong, and it can feel impossible to resist. At those times of high relapse risk, please be very gentle with yourself. Distract yourself with healthy activities and seek healthy social support. And read that list of all of the abusive things that happened to you. If you can ride out the biochemical craving, it should fade. If you can delay negative action during these intense "craving" periods, you can prevent relapse. People who have not dealt with addiction probably do not understand how powerful such feelings can be. They will not understand how overwhelming the drive toward relapse may be. But utilizing these tips should be helpful.

Also, if you are suffering because you cannot stand the idea of the abuser being with someone else, it may be helpful to face this fear through some imagery work. You can imagine what you are afraid of happening—maybe laugh while you imagine it. Play around with this idea of facing your fear, because it can create an opening for healing and overcoming blocks to recovery from addiction. You can be happy with someone else. And you will survive the idea of the abuser having a relationship with someone new. These emotions can be overwhelming but try to allow yourself to feel them. You can begin by facing them for a very short time, allow your nervous system to tolerate the discomfort, and then allow for the discomfort to fade away. You are already making progress by facing your fear, even for a short time. Good luck to anyone going through this type of situation. It can be one of the greatest challenges of your life. It is good to find the positive in anything in life, even the tragic. Gratitude is healing. There is an opportunity for profound personal growth after the tragedy of these relationships.

This issue is obviously very broad, but in general, maximize positive healthy relationships in life and positive social interaction, while protecting against negative and stressful relationships. We need family, friends, community, and social support. We need empathetic political leaders, corporate leaders, and community leaders. Simultaneously, we need to be able to recognize abuse and toxicity with respect to relationships and be able to protect ourselves from that negativity.

Sunshine

To achieve optimal health and well-being, including the prevention and treatment of neurological diseases, sunshine exposure is generally necessary. Human beings were designed to be outside much more than modern lifestyles typically involve. There are negative effects associated with sedentary indoor lifestyles related to lack of exercise, lack of sunshine, and sitting for extended periods of time.

In my opinion, there is a disconnect between the obvious association between disease and vitamin D deficiency on the one hand and on the other hand, the questionable benefit from vitamin D supplementation. There are different issues here that require understanding and consideration. Certainly, vitamin D has a profound role in the human body.

However, it could be that vitamin D status is simply a marker for general sun exposure. While vitamin D production is part of the benefit of sunshine exposure, it certainly is not the only benefit.[1] It would seem wise to advocate maximizing exposure to sunshine in order to maximize benefits with the caution that sunburn must be avoided. There is scientific evidence to support this position.[2] In fact, this evidence demonstrates that sun exposure itself may help prevent Alzheimer's disease, multiple sclerosis, and Parkinson's disease, however, this is not necessarily due to vitamin D production. Lack of sunshine (but again, not necessarily because of the vitamin D issue), is also associated with autism.[3] Besides enhancing vitamin D production, sunshine also benefits the circadian rhythm, nitric oxide, serotonin, melatonin, and the immune system.[4] It should be noted that there is evidence that a lack of sunshine in pregnant women and neonates may increase the risk of schizophrenia in the future for those new-borns.[5-6] Inadequate sunshine in pregnant women may also increase the risk of autism in that child. Further evidence that supports the idea that the effects of lack of sunshine cannot be overcome through simple vitamin D supplementation comes from disappointing results in trials of vitamin D in multiple sclerosis.[7] Taken together, all of this suggests that lack of sunshine increases the risk of neurological conditions. Sunshine exposure should generally be recommended for both prevention and treatment of all neurological conditions, particularly Alzheimer's disease, multiple sclerosis, and Parkinson's disease. There is a very real possibility that vitamin D supplementation may not work as well (if at all) in terms of prevention and treatment of neurological conditions.

Supplementation with vitamin D should be avoided unless absolutely necessary (to be determined on a case-by-case basis based on latitude, weather, ability to be outside, melanin concentration in the skin, and blood levels of vitamin D). It would show a lack of understanding of history to push widespread vitamin D supplementation on the assump-tion that it is safe and efficacious.

Humility in medicine requires trust in the body (to regulate vitamin D production from sunshine and derive maximum benefits with min-imal risk). Overriding that innate wisdom of the body with vitamin D supplementation should not be done carelessly. When supplementation is necessary, it should be in the form of vitamin D3 derived from lichen. This form of vitamin D3 does not contribute to climate change in the same manner as the animal-agriculture-associated, lanolin-based vita-min D3 supplements. The lichen-derived vitamin D3 also has benefits in terms of animal rights when compared to lanolin-derived vitamin

D3. For maximum safety, dosage can be up to 2,000 international units per day.[8-9]

It is also recommended that people avoid night-shift work. This touches on the issues of both sun exposure (which requires being awake during the day) and sleep habits. Night-shift work can worsen epilepsy,[10] and increase multiple sclerosis risk.[11]

People should always avoid getting sunburned. There may also be people with specific health conditions that would prevent them from getting sun exposure. Please consult your healthcare provider to ensure there are no contraindications to regular sun exposure. In cases where sun exposure is not possible, and under healthcare practitioner guidance, vitamin D3 (vegan sourced) can be utilized. Dosage recommendations do vary, and in general, healthy adults with no contraindications may safely use up to 5,000 international units of vitamin D per day. In general, try to get the vitamin D from sunshine first, and only supplement when necessary. Again, it is generally safer to rely on sunshine (between 10am-3pm is the best time), keeping in mind that one should always avoid sunburn and heat stroke. If sunshine is not possible, ask your physician if it is safe for you to utilize vitamin D supplements, and use the lowest possible dosage of vegan vitamin D3. Dosages will vary, and some people may need to take 2,000 IU per day, for example, while others may need 5,000 IU per day. When deciding on this issue of sunshine and vitamin D supplementation, please check your latitude on the planet, as vitamin D production varies by time of day, latitude, and season. Considering your individual health situation along with these factors can facilitate making a proper decision regarding supplementation.

Water-damaged Homes

In today's modern world, the issue of mold and water damage should be addressed. A discussion of neurological and psychological health cannot be complete without giving a broad overview of this issue. There have been many profound changes in the environment since the Industrial Revolution. The use of Benomyl may have led to an increase in the toxicity of mycotoxins produced by mold,[1] which means that today's mold may be more toxin-producing than in the past. In addition, there are issues with the use of building materials which increase the likelihood of illness. Constant high humidity with low airflow (low ventilation) increases the risk of problematic mold in the home. The mold issue is a very broad topic, with many intricacies.[2-3] Mold, combined with the toxins they may produce under specific circumstances, can lead to a variety of neurological and psychological symptoms. Some people are more sensitive to mold. It is very important to address any water damage in the home as quickly as possible. Do not ignore leaking pipes, strange musty smells, etc. Having plants in the house can be beneficial in creating a more natural environment in the home since the separation of the home from nature creates the type of mono-culture environment which can make people ill. It is important to avoid getting stressed about the mold issue, because it is very common. Calmly planning to address the mold issue is the best way forward, maximizing the benefits of avoiding the mycotoxins while simultaneously minimizing stress. Cleaning up water-related accidents within 24 hours minimizes the chances of developing a mold problem. After a problem has already occurred, highly qualified professionals who utilize maximum safety protocols should repair water damage in the home.

CHAPTER 2 REFERENCES

Big Picture Healing:

1. Klinghardt, D. "The 5 Levels of Healing." *Explore.* 2005; 14(4). Accessed August 8, 2023. http://klinghardtacademy.com/images/stories/ 5_levels_of_healing/Klinghardt_Article_5_Levels_of_Healing.pdf.

Confusion, Diagnostic and Therapeutic Issues, and Complexity of Healing Options:

1. Randall-May, C. *Praynow.net.* Published 2023. Accessed September 8, 2023. https:// praynow.net/index.html.

2. "NOMI. NOMI". Accessed September 8, 2023. https://www.nomimedical-intuition. org/.

Environmental Medicine References:

1. Greger, M, and G Stone. *How Not to Die: Discover the Foods Scientifically Proven to Prevent and Reverse Disease.* New York, New York: Flatiron Books; 2015.

2. Erkekoglu, P, and T Baydar. "Acrylamide neurotoxicity." *Nutritional Neuroscience.* 2014; 17(2): 49-57. Doi: 10.1179/1476830513Y.0000000065.

3. "Dutch drinking water is of top quality as shown by international research." *NieuwsberichtenEngels Vewin.* http://www.vewin.nl/english/ News/Paginas/Dutch_drinking_water_is_of_top_quality_as_shown_by_international_research_20.aspx. Accessed January 14, 2019.

4. Carpenter, DO. "Effects of metals on the nervous system of humans and animals." *International Journal of Occupational Medicine and Environmental Health.* 2001; 14(3): 209-218.

5. Chin-Chan, M, J Navarro-Yepes, and B Quintanilla-Vega. "Environmental pollutants as risk factors for neurodegenerative disorders: Alzheimer and Parkinson diseases." *Front Cell Neurosci.* 2015; 9: 124. Published Apr 10, 2015. Doi: 10.3389/fncel.2015.00124.

6. Kianoush, S, M Sadeghi, and M Balali-Mood. "Recent Advances in the Clinical Management of Lead Poisoning." *Acta Medica Iranica.* 2015; 53(6): 327-336.

7. Hardell, L, and C Sage. "Biological effects from electromagnetic field exposure and public exposure standards." *Biomedicine & Pharmacotherapy.* 2008; 62(2): 104-109. Doi: 10.1016/j.biopha.2007.12.004.

8. Children's Health Defense. "Help Children's Health Defense and RFK, Jr. end the epidemic of poor health plaguing our children." *Children's Health Defense.* Published 2019. Accessed August 22, 2023. https://childrenshealthdefense.org/.

9. Yurovsky, S. "FCT Field Control Therapy." *www.yurkovsky.com.* Accessed September 13, 2023. https://www.yurkovsky.com/.

Exercise References:

1. Ahlskog, JE. "Aerobic Exercise: Evidence for a Direct Brain Effect to Slow Parkinson Disease Progression." *Mayo Clinic Proceedings.* 2018; 93(3): 360-372. Doi: 10.1016/j.mayocp.2017.12.015.

2. Bhalsing, KS, MM Abbas, and LCS Tan. "Role of Physical Activity in Parkinson's Disease." *Annals of Indian Academy of Neurology.* 2018; 21(4): 242-249. Doi: 10.4103/aian.AIAN_169_18.

3. Hernández, SS, PF Sandreschi, FCD Silva, et al. "What Are the Benefits of Exercise for Alzheimer's Disease? A Systematic Review of the Past 10 Years." *Journal of Aging and Physical Activity.* 2015; 23(4): 659-668. Doi: 10.1123/japa.2014-0180.

4. Dalgas, U. "Exercise therapy in multiple sclerosis and its effects on function and the brain." *Neurodegenerative Disease Management.* 2017; 7(6s): 35-40. Doi: 10.2217/nmt-2017-0040.

5. Halabchi, F, Z Alizadeh, MA Sahraian, and M Abolhasani. "Exercise prescription for patients with multiple sclerosis; potential benefits and practical recommendations." *BMC Neurology.* 2017; 17(1). Doi: 10.1186/ s12883-017-0960-9.

6. Fritz, NE, AK Rao, D Kegelmeyer, et al. "Physical Therapy and Exercise Interventions in Huntington's Disease: A Mixed Methods Systematic Review." *Journal of Huntington's Disease.* 2017; 6(3): 217-235. Doi: 10.3233/ jhd-170260.

7. Pedersen, BK, and B Saltin. "Exercise as medicine - evidence for prescribing exercise as therapy in 26 different chronic diseases." *Scandinavian Journal of Medicine & Science in Sports.* 2015; 25: 1-72. Doi: 10.1111/ sms.12581.

8. Greger, M, and G Stone. *How Not to Die: Discover the Foods Scientifically Proven to Prevent and Reverse Disease.* New York, New York: Flatiron Books; 2015.

Fasting:

1. Mattson, MP, VD Longo, and M Harvie. "Impact of intermittent fasting on health and disease processes." *Ageing Research Reviews.* 2017; 39: 46-58. Doi: 10.1016/j.arr.2016.10.005.

2. Shelton, HM. *The Science and Fine Arts of Fasting.* Mansfield Centre, CT: Martino Publishing; 2013.

3. Buhner, SH. *The Transformational Power of Fasting: The Way to Spiritual, Physical, and Emotional Rejuvenation.* Rochester, VT: Healing Arts Press; 2012.

4. Lisle, DJ, and A Goldhamer. *The Pleasure Trap: Mastering the Hidden Force That Undermines Health & Happiness.* Summertown, TN: Healthy Living Publications; 2006.

5. Fuhrman, J. *Fasting and Eating for Health: a Medical Doctors Program for Conquering Disease.* New York: St. Martins Griffin; 1995.

6. Fung, J, and J Moore. *The Complete Guide to Fasting: Heal Your Body through Intermittent, Alternate-Day, and Extended Fasting.* Las Vegas: Victory Belt Publishing; 2016.

7. Klaper, M. Fasting: *Safe and Effective Use of an Ancient Healing Therapy.* United States of America: Ruester Productions; 2011. https://www.doctorklaper.com/videos.

8. Goldhamer, A. "Water Fasting Can Save Your Life." https://www.youtube.com/watch? v=QNiGB7EuNvo. Published July 15, 2018. Accessed December 25, 2018.

9. Cott, A. "Controlled Fasting Treatment for Schizophrenia." *Journal of Orthomolecular Medicine.* 1974; 3(4): 301-311. http://www.orthomolecular.org/library/jom/1974/pdf/1974-v03n04-p301.pdf.

Gastrointestinal Health:

1. Gordon, James S. *Transforming Trauma: Discovering Wholeness and Healing after Trauma.* London, Yellow Kite, 2021.

2. Bush, Zach. "Home." *Zachbushmd.com.* Accessed 31 July 2023.

Infectious Agents:

1. Alam, M, Q Alam, M Kamal, et al. "Infectious Agents and Neurodegenerative Diseases: Exploring the Links." *Current Topics in Medicinal Chemistry.* 2017; 17(12): 1390-1399. Doi: 10.2174/1568026617666170103164040.

2. Sochocka, M, K Zwolińska, and J Leszek. "The Infectious Etiology of Alzheimer's Disease." *Curr Neuropharmacol.* 2017; 15(7): 996-1009.

3. Zivadinov, R, Y Guan, D Jakimovski, M Ramanathan, and B Weinstock-Guttman. "The role of Epstein-Barr virus in multiple sclerosis: from molecular pathophysiology to in vivo imaging." *Neural Regeneration Research.* 2019; 14(3): 373-386. Doi: 10.4103/1673-5374.245462.

4. Dardiotis, E, Z Tsouris, A-FA Mentis, et al. "*H. pylori* and Parkinson's disease: Meta-analyses including clinical severity." *Clinical Neurology and Neurosurgery.* 2018; 175: 16-24. Doi: 10.1016/j.clineuro.2018.09.039.

5. Fuglewicz, A, P Piotrowski, and A Stodolak. "Relationship between toxoplasmosis and schizophrenia: A review." *Advances in Clinical and Experimental Medicine.* 2017; 26(6): 1031-1036. Doi: 10.17219/acem/61435.

6. Bransfield, RC. "Neuropsychiatric Lyme Borreliosis: An Overview with a Focus on a Specialty Psychiatrist's Clinical Practice." *Healthcare (Basel).* 2018; 6(3): 104. Published Aug 25, 2018. Doi: 10.3390/healthcare6030104.

7. Feng J, S Zhang, W Shi, N Zubcevik, J Miklossy, and Y Zhang. "Selective Essential Oils from Spice or Culinary Herbs Have High Activity against Stationary Phase and Biofilm." *Borrelia burgdorferi. Front Med (Lausanne).* 2017; 4: 169. Published 2017 Oct 11. Doi: 10.3389/fmed.2017.00169.

8. Feng, J, W Shi, J Miklossy, G Tauxe, C Mcmeniman, and Y Zhang. "Identification of Essential Oils with Strong Activity against Stationary Phase Borrelia burgdorferi." *Antibiotics (Basel, Switzerland).* 2018; 7(4): 89. Doi: 10.3390/antibiotics7040089.

Inner Work:

1. Breggin, Peter R. *Guilt, Shame, and Anxiety.* Prometheus Books, 2014.

2. Peyton, Sarah. *YOUR RESONANT SELF WORKBOOK: From Self-Sabotage to Self-Care.* W W Norton, 2021.

3. Dispenza, Joe. "GOLOV-20 Meditation (Official Video)." Www.youtube.com, 24 Apr. 2020, www.youtube.com/watch?v=FZXVix4TNOI. Accessed 17 July 2023.

4. —. "U•Inspire•Me Meditation (Official Video)." Www.youtube.com, 2 May 2020, www.youtube.com/watch?v=ax7GWg6KQbY. Accessed 17 July 2023.

5. Oprah.com. Oprah.com. https://www.oprah.com/index.html. Accessed August 18, 2023.

6. —. "OWN." YouTube. Accessed August 18, 2023. https://www.youtube.com/@OWN

7. Moorjani, A. *Dying to Be Me: My Journey from Cancer, to near Death, to True Healing, 1st ed.* Hay House; 2012.

8. Lipton, Bruce H., "Home." Accessed September 8, 2023. https://www.brucelipton.com/

9. PSYCH-K Centre International. *Psych-k.com.* Published 2019. Accessed November 5, 2019. https://psych-k.com/

Mind-Body Medicine:

1. Ornish, D. *Dr. Dean Ornish's Program for Reversing Heart Disease.* New York, NY: Ballantine Books; 1991.

2. Murray, MT, and JE Pizzorno. *The Encyclopedia of Natural Medicine, 3rd ed.* New York, NY: Atria Paperback (Simon & Schuster); 2012.

Nutrition:

1. Montgomery, BD. *The Food Prescription for Better Health: a Cardiologist's Proven Method to Reverse Heart Disease, Diabetes, Obesity, and Other Chronic Illnesses, Naturally!* Houston, TX: Delworth Pub.; 2011.

2. Fuhrman, J. *Fasting and Eating for Health: a Medical Doctors Program for Conquering Disease.* New York: St. Martins Griffin; 1995.

3. Lisle, DJ, and A Goldhamer. *The Pleasure Trap: Mastering the Hidden Force That Undermines Health & Happiness.* Summertown, TN: Healthy Living Publications; 2006.

4. Esselstyn, CB. *Prevent and Reverse Heart Disease: The Revolutionary, Scientifically Proven, Nutrition-Based Cure.* New York, NY: Avery (Penguin Group); 2008.

5. Ornish, D. *Dr. Dean Ornish's Program for Reversing Heart Disease.* New York, NY: Ballantine Books; 1991.

6. McDougall, JA, and M McDougall. *The Starch Solution: Eat the Foods You Love, Regain Your Health, and Lose the Weight for Good!* New York, NY: Rodale; 2012.

7. Barnard, ND. *Power Foods for the Brain: an Effective 3-Step Plan to Protect Your Mind and Strengthen Your Memory.* Grand Central Pub; 2014.

8. Greger, M, and G Stone. *How Not to Die: Discover the Foods Scientifically Proven to Prevent and Reverse Disease.* New York, New York: Flatiron Books; 2015.

9. NutritionFacts.org. "Acrylamide." https://nutritionfacts.org/topics/ acrylamide/. Accessed December 26, 2018.

10. —. "Advanced Glycation End-products (AGEs)." https://nutrition-facts.org/topics/advanced-glycation-end-products/. Accessed December 26, 2018.

11. Shah, SP, and JE Duda. "Dietary modifications in Parkinson's disease: A neuroprotective intervention?" *Medical Hypotheses.* 2015; 85(6): 1002-1005. Doi: 10.1016/j.mehy.2015.08.01.

12. Hughes, KC, X Gao, IY Kim, et al. "Intake of dairy foods and risk of Parkinson's disease." *Neurology.* 2017; 89(1): 46-52. Doi: 10.1212/ wnl.0000000000004057.

13. Baroni, L, C Bonetto, F Tessan, et al. "Pilot dietary study with normoproteic protein-redistributed plant-food diet and motor performance in patients with Parkinson's disease." *Nutritional Neuroscience.* 2011; 14(1): 1-9. Doi: 10.1179/174313211x12 966635733231.

14. Swank, RL. "Multiple sclerosis: fat-oil relationship." *Nutrition.* 1991; 7(5): 368-376.

15. Yadav, V, G Marracci, E Kim, et al. "Low-fat, plant-based diet in multiple sclerosis: A randomized controlled trial." *Multiple Sclerosis and Related Disorders.* 2016; 9: 80-90. Doi: 10.1016/j.msard.2016.07.001.

16. Patel, H, S Chandra, S Alexander, J Soble, and KA Williams. "Plant-Based Nutrition: An Essential Component of Cardiovascular Disease Prevention and Management." *Current Cardiology Reports.* 2017; 19(10). Doi: 10.1007/ s11886-017-0909-z.

17. Najjar, RS, CE Moore, and BD Montgomery. "A defined, plant-based diet utilized in an outpatient cardiovascular clinic effectively treats hypercholesterolemia and hypertension and reduces medications." *Clinical Cardiology.* 2018; 41(3): 307-313. Doi: 10.1002/clc.22863.

18. Esselstyn, CB. "Defining an Overdue Requiem for Palliative Cardiovascular Medicine." *American Journal of Lifestyle Medicine.* 2016; 10(5): 313-317. Doi: 10.1177/1559827616638647.

19. Esselstyn, CB, G Gendy, J Doyle, M Golubic, and MF Roizen. "A way to reverse CAD?" *The Journal of Family Practice.* 2014; 63(7): 356-364b.

20. Esselstyn, CB. "Resolving the Coronary Artery Disease Epidemic Through Plant-Based Nutrition." *Preventive Cardiology.* 2001; 4(4): 171-177. Doi: 10.1111/j.1520-037x.2001.00538.x.

21. —. "In cholesterol lowering, moderation kills." *Cleveland Clinic Journal of Medicine.* 2000; 67(8): 560-564. Doi: 10.3949/ccjm.67.8.560.

22. Ornish, D, S Brown, J Billings, et al. "Can lifestyle changes reverse coronary heart disease?" *The Lancet.* 1990; 336(8708): 129-133. Doi: 10.1016/0140-6736(90)91656-u.

23. Goodland, R, and J Anhang. "Livestock and Climate Change: What if the key actors in climate change are...cows, pigs, and chickens?" *World Watch.* 2009: 10-19.

24. Factory Farms. "A Well-Fed World." https://awfw.org/factory-farms/. Accessed December 26, 2018.

25. Greger, M. "When Meat Can Be a Lifesaver | NutritionFacts.org." Published May 2, 2012. Accessed August 23, 2023. https://nutritionfacts.org/ video/when-meat-can-be-a-lifesaver/.

26. Mills, Milton. "The Comparative Anatomy of Eating." https://drmiltonmillsplant-basednation.com/the-comparative-anatomy-of-eating/.

27. Klaper, Michael. "Physician, Speaker, Educator." Published 2013. Accessed August 30, 2023. https://www.doctorklaper.com/.

28. — YouTube playlist. Accessed August 30, 2023. https://www.youtube.com/@DoctorKlaper.

29. —. "Meat Cravings - Managing Meat Cravings When Switching To A Plant-Based Diet." Accessed August 30, 2023. https://www.youtube.com/ watch?v=5gffthGIfPs.

Raising Children:

1. Neufeld, Gordon, and Gabor Maté. *Hold on to Your Kids: Why Parents Need to Matter More than Peers.* 2004. Vintage Canada ed., Toronto, Vintage Canada, 2005.

2. Maté, Gabor, and Daniel Maté. *The Myth of Normal: Trauma, Illness, and Healing in a Toxic Culture.* London, Vermillion, 2022.

Relationships and Health:

1. Maté, Gabor, and Daniel Maté. *The Myth of Normal: Trauma, Illness, and Healing in a Toxic Culture.* London, Vermillion, 2022.

2. Durvasula, Ramani. *Don't You Know Who I Am?: How to Stay Sane in an Era of Narcissism, Entitlement, and Incivility.* New York Nashville, Post Hill Press, 2019.

3. —. *Should I Stay or Should I Go?: Surviving a Relationship with a Narcissist.* New York Nashville, Post Hill Press, 2015.

4. —"DoctorRamani - YouTube." www.youtube.com/@DoctorRamani.

Sunshine:

1. Rhee, HVD, JW Coebergh, and ED Vries. "Is prevention of cancer by sun exposure more than just the effect of vitamin D? A systematic review of epidemiological studies." *European Journal of Cancer.* 2013; 49(6): 1422-1436. Doi: 10.1016/j.ejca.2012.11.001.

2. Iacopetta, K, LE Collins-Praino, FTA Buisman-Pijlman, J Liu, AD Hutchinson, and MR Hutchinson. "Are the protective benefits of vitamin D in neurodegenerative disease dependent on route of administration? A systematic review." *Nutritional Neuroscience.* September 2018: 1-30. Doi: 10.1080/1028415x.2018.1493807.

3. Hoel, D, and FD Gruijl. "Sun Exposure Public Health Directives." *International Journal of Environmental Research and Public Health.* 2018; 15(12): 2794. Doi: 10.3390/ijerph15122794.

4. Rhee, HVD, ED Vries, and J Coebergh. "Regular sun exposure benefits health." *Medical Hypotheses.* 2016; 97: 34-37. Doi: 10.1016/ j.mehy.2016.10.011.

5. Anjum, I, SS Jaffery, M Fayyaz, Z Samoo, and S Anjum. "The Role of Vitamin D in Brain Health: A Mini Literature Review." *Cureus.* October 2018. Doi: 10.7759/cureus.2960.

6. Eyles, DW, M Trzaskowski, AAE Vinkhuyzen, et al. "The association between neonatal vitamin D status and risk of schizophrenia." *Scientific Reports.* 2018; 8(1). Doi: 10.1038/s41598-018-35418-z 7.

7. Jagannath, VA, G Filippini, C Di Pietrantonj, et al. "Vitamin D for the management of multiple sclerosis." *The Cochrane Database of Systematic Reviews.* September 2018. Doi: 10.1002/14651858.CD008422.pub3.

8. Esselstyn, CB. *Prevent and Reverse Heart Disease: The Revolutionary, Scientifically Proven, Nutrition-Based Cure.* New York, NY: Avery (Penguin Group); 2008.

9. Greger, M, and G Stone. *How Not to Die: Discover the Foods Scientifically Proven to Prevent and Reverse Disease.* New York, New York: Flatiron Books; 2015.

10. LaDou, J. "Health effects of shift work." *The Western Journal of Medicine.* 1982; 137(6): 525-530.

11. Gustavsen, S, H Søndergaard, D Oturai, et al. "Shift work at young age is associated with increased risk of multiple sclerosis in a Danish population." *Multiple Sclerosis and Related Disorders.* 2016; 9: 104-109. Doi: 10.1016/ j.msard.2016.06.010.

Water Damaged Homes:

1. Shoemaker, RC. *Surviving Mold: Life in the Era of Dangerous Buildings.* Otter Bay Books, LLC; 2010.

2. Nathan, N. *Toxic.* Victory Belt Publishing; 2018.

3. Crista J. *Break the Mold: 5 Tools to Conquer Mold and Take Back Your Health.* Wellness Ink Publishing; 2018.

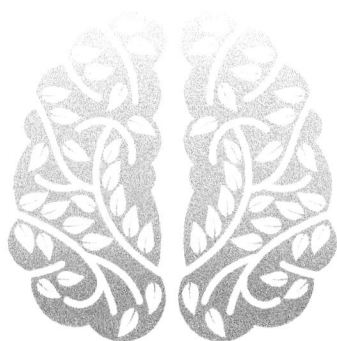

CHAPTER 3

Conditions

Addiction

The foundation for addiction treatment should be addressing any potential trauma. Therefore, please refer to the "Post-Traumatic Stress Disorder" entry in this chapter for details on treating trauma, PTSD, and Complex PTSD. Please follow the general nutrition and exercise recommendations discussed in this work. Also vital are the sections on Inner Work and Big Picture Healing (in Chapter 2). Finding social support, connection, and meaning in life is vital with addiction treatment, and in general. The section "Policies on Addiction and Criminal Justice" in Chapter 4 is also important. Please address any coexisting mental health conditions in addition to the addiction.

Aerotoxic Syndrome

The neurological and psychological impacts of flying are important, and often ignored issues. In my personal experience, the neuropsychological impact of flying has been quite significant. There is something particularly non-physiologic about flying as a mode of transportation. Of course, the issue of climate change and flying is also significant and also supports the case that flying should be minimized as much as possible. There are significant practical issues involved here, but in general, it is best to minimize flying for both health and environmental reasons. Alternative modes of transportation should be used whenever possible, and people should consider the negative impact of air travel before making career and educational choices that take them far from home and family. Minimizing, and preferably eliminating, private jets that consume fossil fuels would be a wise policy. And the idea of flying for vacations must be reconsidered for the sake of our planet's future, on which our survival depends. Flying to see family certainly seems more justifiable than flying for tourism purposes, but both should be minimized. One certainly hopes that rapid transportation (including electric or sustainable aviation and high-speed rail) which does not rely on fossil fuels will soon become widely available. In the meantime, keep air travel to a minimum.

In terms of the health impacts of flying, there are numerous issues. Jet lag is well-known and obviously negative in terms of neurological function. Sleep deprivation can be associated with flying. In addition to jet lag and sleep deprivation, there are issues of relative oxygen deprivation, rapid air pressure changes, and ionizing radiation from high altitudes. Dehydration can also be an issue that impacts people traveling by air.

Exposure to toxic cabin air may also cause a wide variety of neurological and psychological health effects.[1-2] In essence, a design flaw sometimes allows toxic chemicals to leak into the cabin air. It is a very serious issue that can cause disability in extreme circumstances. Negative cognitive, neurological, and psychological symptoms may be related to this toxic exposure. Aerotoxic syndrome is very serious. Prevention would ideally involve not flying. If this is not practical, flying only on Boeing 787 aircraft will virtually eliminate the risk of toxic exposure, as the design flaw referred to above has been corrected in these planes, making the cabin air quality far safer than in other aircraft. It is possible to find routes with selected aircraft (for example, Boeing 787) using www.flightsfrom.com, and this can be very useful to protect neurological health.[3] The Boeing 787 also has other health advantages, including less noise pollution and less hypoxia (low oxygen) for passengers.[4]

Easy Jet has moved in the right direction on this issue of toxic cabin air.[5] Their customer service confirmed to me that their entire fleet now has carbon filtration.[6] However, at the time of this writing, their fleet does not utilize the Boeing 787.[7] Thus, the first choice would be to not fly. The second choice would be using the Boeing 787 aircraft (which is utilized by different airlines). Easy Jet is likely an improvement over the average experience in terms of the health impacts of flying, but in my experience, the Boeing 787 is a healthier option.

Using a mask with a carbon filter, such as one produced by Cambridge Mask Company,[8] is a good idea if you are unable to fly on a Boeing 787. If you're on a plane with this design flaw regarding cabin air quality, using such a mask can reduce risk, particularly during turbulence, take-off, landing, or if there are any strange smells of exhaust or other odors.

Neurofeedback may be beneficial in treating Aerotoxic Syndrome.[9] However, please refer to the discussion on neurofeedback in the "Trauma Healing" section of this chapter for possible limitations in its effectiveness. I would expect that fasting may have utility in treating Aerotoxic Syndrome, but please refer to the "Fasting" section in Chapter 2 for precautions and contraindications. The general lifestyle recommendations discussed elsewhere in this work should be beneficial as well.

Alzheimer's Disease and Dementia

Eat a 100% whole-food organic plant-based diet with supplemental vitamin B12. Eliminate artificial colors, flavors, and preservatives. Eliminate trans fats. Eliminate added salt, oil, and sugar. Food intake should be derived as much as possible from raw, boiled, or steamed food while keeping high-temperature cooking (baking, frying) to a minimum. Avoiding high-temperature cooking minimizes exposure to acrylamide (a neurotoxin).

Ensure optimal sunshine exposure (but avoid sunburn). Avoid shift work. Consider water-only fasting, which may be profoundly useful (see "Fasting" section above for precautions/contraindications). Ensure adequate and appropriate physical activity. Eat 100% organic and live an organic and ecological lifestyle to minimize exposure to toxins (including neurotoxins). Avoid lead (old paint, water piping, etc.) and mercury (dental amalgam, fish, coal-burning power plants, broken fluorescent light bulbs, old thermometers, etc.).

Minimize exposure to electromagnetic fields. Avoid cellphone use. Avoid wireless telephones. Utilize corded landlines and wired internet cables and routers. If cellphone use is necessary, keep it at a maximum distance from the body and use the speaker. Keep general technology use to a minimum. Minimize technology in the bedroom and keep electromagnetic field exposure as low as possible. Addressing issues related to Mind-Body Medicine, including stress management, positive thinking, increasing social support, healing past trauma, prayer, and spirituality, may be beneficial.

The following plants may have utility in Alzheimer's Disease: *Allium sativum, Bacopa monnieri, Brassica oleracea, Camelia sinensis, Centella asiatica, Chamaemelum nobile or Matricaria chamomilla, Cinnamomum verum,*

Crocus sativus, Curcuma longa, Ginkgo biloba, Hericium erinaceus, Hypericum perforatum, Nigella sativa, Phyllanthus emblica, Punica granatum, Rosmarinus officinalis, Scutellaria baicalensis, Syzygium aromaticum, Vaccinium myrtillus, Zingiber officinale.

Please refer to the individual herb listings and the other mentioned sections of this work for details, references, and important precautions.

Amyotrophic Lateral Sclerosis (Lou Gehrig's disease)

Eat a 100% whole-food organic plant-based diet with supplemental vitamin B12. Eliminate artificial colors, flavors, and preservatives. Eliminate trans fats. Eliminate added salt, oil, and sugar. Food intake should be derived as much as possible from raw, boiled, or steamed food while keeping high-temperature cooking (baking, frying) to a minimum. Avoiding high-temperature cooking minimizes exposure to acrylamide (a neurotoxin).

Ensure optimal sunshine exposure (but avoid sunburn). Avoid shift work. Water-only fasting may not be advisable with amyotrophic lateral sclerosis. While generally beneficial and theoretically useful for this condition, it is possible that fasting may be harmful with this disease and therefore maximum caution is advised. Ensure adequate and appropriate physical activity based on the individual health situation. Eat 100% organic and live an organic and ecological lifestyle to minimize exposure to toxins (including neurotoxins). Avoid lead (old paint, water piping, etc.) and mercury (dental amalgam, fish, coal-burning power plants, broken fluorescent light bulbs, old thermometers, etc.).

Minimize exposure to electromagnetic fields. Avoid cellphone use. Avoid wireless telephones. Utilize corded landlines and wired internet cables and routers. If cellphone use is necessary, keep it at a maximum distance from the body and use the phone's speaker. Keep general technology use to a minimum. Minimize technology in the bedroom and keep electromagnetic field exposure as low as possible. Addressing issues related to Mind-Body Medicine, including stress management, positive thinking, increasing social support, healing past trauma, prayer, and spirituality may be beneficial. Please see the work of Dr. Gabor Maté for details on the link between repressed anger and ALS. Learning to set boundaries and the healthy expression of anger is vital in the prevention and treatment of ALS.

The following plants may have utility in amyotrophic lateral sclerosis: *Allium sativum, Bacopa monnieri, Brassica oleracea, Camelia sinensis, Centella asiatica, Chamaemelum nobile* or *Matricaria chamomilla, Cinnamomum verum, Curcuma longa, Hericium erinaceus, Hypericum perforatum, Nigella sativa, Phyllanthus emblica, Punica granatum, Rosmarinus officinalis, Scutellaria baicalensis, Vaccinium myrtillus, Zingiber officinale.*

Please refer to the individual herb listings and other mentioned sections of this work for details, references, and important precautions.

Anxiety

Eat a 100% whole-food organic plant-based diet with supplemental vitamin B12. Eliminate artificial colors, flavors, and preservatives. Eliminate trans fats. Eliminate added salt, oil, and sugar. Food intake should be derived as much as possible from raw, boiled, or steamed food while keeping high-temperature cooking (baking, frying) to a minimum. Avoiding high temperature cooking minimizes exposure to acrylamide (a neurotoxin).

Ensure optimal sunshine exposure (but avoid sunburn). Avoid shift work. Consider water-only fasting, which may be useful (see "Fasting" section above for precautions/contraindications). Ensure adequate and appropriate physical activity based on the individual health situation. Eat 100% organic and live an organic and ecological lifestyle to minimize exposure to toxins (including neurotoxins). Avoid lead (old paint, water piping, etc.) and mercury (dental amalgam, fish, coal-burning power plants, broken fluorescent light bulbs, old thermometers, etc.).

Minimize exposure to electromagnetic fields. Avoid cellphone use. Avoid wireless telephones. Utilize corded landlines and wired internet cables. Utilize wired internet routers. If cellphone use is necessary keep it at a maximum distance from the body and use the phone's speaker. Keep general technology use to a minimum. Minimize technology in the bedroom and keep electromagnetic field exposure as low as possible. Addressing issues related to Mind-Body Medicine including stress management, positive thinking, increasing social support, healing past trauma, prayer, and spirituality may be beneficial. Unresolved past trauma and adverse childhood events may be an underlying source of anxiety. Please see the specific section on PTSD below, as it may be very relevant to treating anxiety.

The following plants may have utility in anxiety: *Bacopa monnieri, Chamaemelum nobile* or *Matricaria chamomilla, Hypericum perforatum, Nepeta cataria, Nigella sativa, Passiflora spp., Piper methysticum, Scutellaria baicalensis, Scutellaria lateriflora, Valeriana officinalis.*

Please refer to the individual herb listings and other mentioned sections of this work for details, references, and important precautions.

Autism

Eat a 100% whole-food organic plant-based diet with supplemental vitamin B12. Eliminate artificial colors, flavors, and preservatives. Eliminate trans fats. Eliminate added salt, oil, and sugar. Food intake should be derived as much as possible from raw, boiled, or steamed food while keeping high-temperature cooking (baking, frying) to a minimum. Avoiding high-temperature cooking minimizes exposure to acrylamide (a neurotoxin).

Ensure optimal sunshine exposure (but avoid sunburn). Avoid shift work. Consider water-only fasting for autistic adults, which should be profoundly useful (see "Fasting" section above for precautions/contraindications). Fasting is typically contraindicated in children, although perhaps under specific circumstances very short and medically-supervised fasting may be justifiable. The benefits would have to substantially outweigh the risks in order to justify such an action. I am not making any recommendations with respect to this issue of fasting in autistic children, as again, fasting is generally only utilized in adults. Ensure adequate and appropriate physical activity based on the individual health situation. Eat 100% organic and live an organic and ecological lifestyle to minimize exposure to toxins (including neurotoxins). Avoid lead (old paint, water pipes, etc.) and mercury (dental amalgam, fish, coal-burning power plants, broken fluorescent light bulbs, old thermometers, etc.).

Minimize exposure to electromagnetic fields. Avoid cellphone use. Avoid wireless telephones. Utilize corded landlines and wired internet and routers. If cellphone use is necessary keep it at a maximum distance from the body and use the phone's speaker. Keep general technology use to a minimum. Minimize technology in the bedroom and keep electromagnetic field exposure as low as possible.

Addressing issues related to Mind-Body Medicine including stress management, positive thinking, increasing social support, healing past trauma, prayer, and spirituality may be beneficial.

The following plants may have utility in autism: *Allium sativum, Bacopa monnieri, Brassica oleracea, Camelia sinensis, Centella asiatica, Chamaemelum nobile or Matricaria chamomilla, Cinnamomum verum, Curcuma longa, Ginkgo biloba, Hericium erinaceus, Hypericum perforatum, Nigella sativa, Phyllanthus emblica, Punica granatum, Scutellaria baicalensis, Vaccinium myrtillus, Zingiber officinale.*

Please refer to the individual herb listings and other mentioned sections of this work for details, references, and important precautions.

Brain Fog, Dissociation, Functional Neurological Disorders, and Psychogenic Illness

Dissociation and all dissociation-related symptoms, including depersonalization and derealization, may be caused by trauma.[1] Dissociation is a feeling of disconnection from the body, the feeling of being separated from your life as if your life is not real. A person may feel that their waking life is nothing but a dream. These types of symptoms can be disabling and destroy a person's quality of life. Please refer to the "Post-Traumatic Stress Disorder" section to maximize the chances of recovering from these symptoms.

Functional neurological disorders can include any number of symptoms that are less structural and more functional in terms of what is happening in the nervous system.[2] The symptoms are real and can be disabling. The symptoms are not under the person's voluntary control. This category is extremely broad and can include many issues which are not yet fully understood by modern medicine. One potential cause of functional neurological disorders is psychogenic. That is, the subconscious can, in response to trauma, stress, or repressed emotions, create real physical symptoms in the body as a distraction from the underlying psychological issue.[3] The work of Dr. John E. Sarno offers very valuable guidance in overcoming such issues. In essence, when a person becomes aware that the subconscious is doing this, the created symptoms dissipate. A comprehensive psychotherapy program that addresses past traumas, stress management, and living an authentic life may be very helpful with functional neurological disorders, and in general, as well. Please see the Post-Traumatic Stress Disorder (Trauma Healing including for PTSD and Complex PTSD) section for further details.

Distinguishing between brain fog, cognitive difficulties, and dissociation can be challenging. In my experience, brain fog can mean different things to different people. The recommendations throughout this work aim to maximize mental clarity and reintegration into one's body (healing trauma) by addressing both physical and psychological contributors to neuropsychological health. As a consequence, it is hoped that people with brain fog will see benefits. Extensive neuropsychological testing may be useful for diagnostic purposes. But there can be overlap and vagueness in terms of understanding and naming what is actually happening. Regardless of the exact diagnosis, hopefully, the recommendations here will help maximize neurological and psychological health.

COVID-19 Related Neurological and Psychiatric Issues

The issue of COVID-19 cannot be avoided in a work on neuropsychiatric health. Personally, this virus profoundly impacted my brain. These symptoms took weeks to recede. Dissociation may be worsened by COVID-19. Cognitive impairment certainly may occur. These symptoms can be disabling and very disturbing. The overall recommendations throughout this work should be beneficial in the case of COVID-19-related neuropsychiatric issues.

Please refer to the *Spike Protein Detox Guide* from the World Council for Health for more details on treatment ideas related to COVID-19.[1] While there are many treatment ideas presented in the *Spike Protein Detox Guide*, I want to draw particular attention to sauna use, fasting, vitamin C, vitamin D3 (please use a plant-based form), turmeric (*Curcuma longa*), and *Nigella sativa* as excellent potential options for dealing with COVID-19 related issues. Please consult with a qualified healthcare practitioner before using any of these treatments to ensure safety based on any underlying health conditions and to avoid harmful drug/supplement interactions. If safe use is possible, a healthcare practitioner can also help determine the proper dosage for safety and efficacy. There are precautions and safety issues associated with saunas and fasting, and healthcare provider guidance maximizes safety. I also recommend referring to the sections in this work on fasting, turmeric (*Curcuma longa),* and *Nigella sativa* for more information.

Depression

Eat a 100% whole-food organic plant-based diet with supplemental vitamin B12. Eliminate artificial colors, flavors, and preservatives. Eliminate trans fats. Eliminate added salt, oil, and sugar. Food intake should be derived as much as possible from raw, boiled, or steamed food while keeping high-temperature cooking (baking, frying) to a minimum. Avoiding high-temperature cooking minimizes exposure to acrylamide (a neurotoxin).

Ensure optimal sunshine exposure (but avoid sunburn). Avoid shift work. Consider water-only fasting, which may be profoundly useful (see "Fasting" section above for precautions/contraindications). Ensure adequate and appropriate physical activity based on the individual health situation. Eat 100% organic and live an organic and ecological lifestyle to minimize exposure to toxins (including neurotoxins). Avoid lead (old paint, water piping, etc.) and mercury (dental amalgam, fish, coal-burning power plants, broken fluorescent light bulbs, old ther-mometers, etc.).

Minimize exposure to electromagnetic fields. Avoid cellphone use. Avoid wireless telephones. Utilize corded landlines and wired internet cables and routers. If cellphone use is necessary, keep it at a maximum distance from the body and use the phone's speaker. Keep general technology use to a minimum. Minimize technology in the bedroom and keep electromagnetic field exposure as low as possible.

Addressing issues related to Mind-Body Medicine including stress management, positive thinking, increasing social support, healing past trauma, prayer, and spirituality may be beneficial.

The following plants may have utility in depression: *Bacopa monnieri, Brassica oleracea, Camelia sinensis, Centella asiatica, Chamaemelum nobile* or *Matricaria chamomilla, Cinnamomum verum, Crocus sativus, Curcuma longa, Ginkgo biloba, Hericium erinaceus, Hypericum perforatum, Nigella sativa, Phyllanthus emblica, Punica granatum, Rosmarinus officinalis, Scutellaria baicalensis, Vaccinium myrtillus, Valeriana officinalis, Zingiber officinale.*

Please refer to the individual herb listings and other mentioned sections of this work for details, references, and important precautions.

Epilepsy

Eat a 100% whole-food organic plant-based diet with supplemental vitamin B12. Eliminate artificial colors, flavors, and preservatives. Eliminate trans fats. Eliminate added salt, oil, and sugar. Food intake should be derived as much as possible from raw, boiled, or steamed food while keeping high-temperature cooking (baking, frying) to a minimum. Avoiding high-temperature cooking minimizes exposure to acrylamide (a neurotoxin).

Ensure optimal sunshine exposure (but avoid sunburn). Avoid shift work. Consider water-only fasting, which may be profoundly useful (see "Fasting" section above for precautions/contraindications). Ensure adequate and appropriate physical activity based on the individual health situation. Eat 100% organic and live an organic and ecological lifestyle to minimize exposure to toxins (including neurotoxins). Avoid lead (old paint, water piping, etc.) and mercury (dental amalgam, fish, coal-burning power plants, broken fluorescent light bulbs, old thermometers, etc.).

Minimize exposure to electromagnetic fields. Avoid cellphone use. Avoid wireless telephones. Utilize corded landlines and wired internet cables and routers. If cellphone use is necessary, keep it at a maximum distance from the body and use the phone's speaker. Keep general technology use to a minimum. Minimize technology in the bedroom and keep electromagnetic field exposure as low as possible.

Addressing issues related to Mind-Body Medicine including stress management, positive thinking, increasing social support, healing past trauma, prayer, and spirituality may be beneficial.

The following plants may have utility in epilepsy: *Allium sativum, Bacopa monnieri, Brassica oleracea, Centella asiatica, Chamaemelum nobile or Matricaria chamomilla, Cinnamomum verum, Crocus sativus, Curcuma longa, Hericium erinaceus, Nepeta cataria, Nigella sativa, Passiflora spp., Phyllanthus emblica, Piper methysticum, Punica granatum, Scutellaria baicalensis, Scutellaria lateriflora, Vaccinium myrtillus, Valeriana officinalis.*

Please refer to the individual herb listings and other mentioned sections of this work for details, references, and important precautions.

Huntington's Chorea

Eat a 100% whole-food organic plant-based diet with supplemental vitamin B12. Eliminate artificial colors, flavors, and preservatives. Eliminate trans fats. Eliminate added salt, oil, and sugar. Food intake should be derived as much as possible from raw, boiled, or steamed food while keeping high-temperature cooking (baking, frying) to a minimum. Avoiding high-temperature cooking minimizes exposure to acrylamide (a neurotoxin).

Ensure optimal sunshine exposure (but avoid sunburn). Avoid shift work. Consider water-only fasting, which may be profoundly useful (see "Fasting" section above for precautions/contraindications). Ensure adequate and appropriate physical activity based on the individual health situation. Eat 100% organic and live an organic and ecological lifestyle to minimize exposure to toxins (including neurotoxins). Avoid lead (old paint, water piping, etc.) and mercury (dental amalgam, fish, coal-burning power plants, broken fluorescent light bulbs, old thermometers, etc.).

Minimize exposure to electromagnetic fields. Avoid cellphone use. Avoid wireless telephones. Utilize corded landlines and wired internet cables and routers. If cellphone use is necessary keep it at a maximum distance from the body and use the phone's speaker. Keep general technology use to a minimum. Minimize technology in the bedroom and keep electromagnetic field exposure as low as possible.

Addressing issues related to Mind-Body Medicine including stress management, positive thinking, increasing social support, healing past trauma, prayer, and spirituality may be beneficial.

The following plants may have utility in Huntington's Chorea: *Allium sativum, Bacopa monnieri, Brassica oleracea, Camelia sinensis, Centella asiatica, Chamaemelum nobile or Matricaria chamomilla, Cinnamomum verum, Curcuma longa, Ginkgo biloba, Hericium erinaceus, Hypericum perforatum, Nigella sativa, Phyllanthus emblica, Punica granatum, Rosmarinus officinalis, Scutellaria baicalensis, Scutellaria lateriflora, Vaccinium myrtillus, Zingiber officinale.*

Please refer to the individual herb listings and other mentioned sections of this work for details, references, and important precautions.

Insomnia

Eat a 100% whole-food organic plant-based diet with supplemental vitamin B12. Eliminate artificial colors, flavors, and preservatives. Eliminate trans fats. Eliminate added salt, oil, and sugar. Food intake should be derived as much as possible from raw, boiled, or steamed food while keeping high-temperature cooking (baking, frying) to a minimum. Avoiding high-temperature cooking minimizes exposure to acrylamide (a neurotoxin).

Ensure optimal sunshine exposure (but avoid sunburn). Avoid shift work. Consider water-only fasting, which may be profoundly useful (see specific section above for precautions/contraindications). Ensure adequate and appropriate physical activity based on the individual health situation. Eat 100% organic and live an organic and ecological lifestyle to minimize exposure to toxins (including neurotoxins). Avoid lead (old paint, water piping, etc.) and mercury (dental amalgam, fish, coal-burning power plants, broken fluorescent light bulbs, old thermometers, etc.).

Minimize exposure to electromagnetic fields. Avoid cellphone use. Avoid wireless telephones. Utilize corded landlines and wired internet cables and routers. If cellphone use is necessary keep it at a maximum distance from the body and use the phone's speaker. Keep general technology use to a minimum. Minimize technology in the bedroom and keep electromagnetic field exposure as low as possible.

Addressing issues related to Mind-Body Medicine including stress management, positive thinking, increasing social support, healing past trauma, prayer, and spirituality may be beneficial. For insomnia related to trauma, please refer to the section on Post-Traumatic Stress Disorder.

The following plants may have utility in insomnia: *Chamaemelum nobile* or *Matricaria chamomilla, Hypericum perforatum, Nepeta cataria, Nigella sativa, Passiflora spp., Piper methysticum, Scutellaria baicalensis, Scutellaria lateriflora, Valeriana officinalis.*

Please refer to the individual herb listings and other mentioned sections of this work for details, references, and important precautions.

Multiple Sclerosis

Eat a 100% whole-food organic plant-based diet with supplemental vitamin B12. Eliminate artificial colors, flavors, and preservatives. Eliminate trans fats. Eliminate added salt, oil, and sugar. Food intake should be derived as much as possible from raw, boiled, or steamed food while keeping high-temperature cooking (baking, frying) to a minimum. Avoiding high-temperature cooking minimizes exposure to acrylamide (a neurotoxin).

Ensure optimal sunshine exposure (but avoid sunburn). Avoid shift work. Consider water-only fasting, which may be profoundly useful (see specific section above for precautions/contraindications). Ensure adequate and appropriate physical activity based on the individual health situation. Eat 100% organic and live an organic and ecological lifestyle to minimize exposure to toxins (including neurotoxins). Avoid lead (old paint, water piping, etc.) and mercury (dental amalgam, fish, coal-burning power plants, broken fluorescent light bulbs, old thermometers, etc.).

Minimize exposure to electromagnetic fields. Avoid cellphone use. Avoid wireless telephones. Utilize corded landlines and wired internet cables. Utilize wired internet routers. If cellphone use is necessary, keep it at a maximum distance from the body and use the phone's speaker. Keep general technology use to a minimum. Minimize technology in the bedroom, and keep electromagnetic field exposure as low as possible.

Addressing issues related to Mind-Body Medicine including stress management, positive thinking, increasing social support, healing past trauma, prayer, and spirituality may be beneficial.

The following plants may have utility in Multiple Sclerosis: *Allium sativum, Bacopa monnieri, Brassica oleracea, Camelia sinensis, Centella asiatica, Chamaemelum nobile* or *Matricaria chamomilla, Cinnamomum verum, Curcuma longa, Ginkgo biloba, Hericium erinaceus, Hypericum perforatum, Nepeta cataria, Nigella sativa, Passiflora spp., Phyllanthus emblica, Piper methysticum, Punica granatum, Rosmarinus officinalis, Scutellaria baicalensis, Scutellaria lateriflora, Syzygium aromaticum, Vaccinium myrtillus, Valeriana officinalis, Zingiber officinale.*

Please refer to the individual herb listings and other sections of this work for details, references, and important precautions.

Obsessive-Compulsive Disorder (OCD)

I have significant personal experience with this issue. Cognitive behavioral therapy (CBT) is often recommended in treating OCD. If the compulsions are observable and preventable (example: handwashing), CBT is likely to be more successful. If the compulsions are internal and non-observable (mentally checking, for example), it may be difficult to prevent the mental process compulsion. This can make CBT treatment less successful.

Other treatments can sometimes bring the OCD under control and allow the CBT to become more useful, particularly for internal compulsions. Please refer to the "Infectious Agents" section for information related to Lyme Disease and OCD.

Kundalini Yoga may be beneficial for obsessive-compulsive disorder.[1-2] Specifically, a technique that involves covering the right nostril with the right thumb and breaking up the 4 sections of breathing (in, hold, out, hold) into even components in terms of time, is a core technique in the Kundalini Yoga treatment of OCD. The eventual goal is to practice this technique 31 minutes per day, with 15 seconds per segment of the breath (15 seconds in, 15 seconds hold, 15 seconds out, 15 seconds hold). I personally have found this type of nostril breathing to be extremely helpful.

Psilocybin may have utility in the treatment of obsessive-compulsive disorder.[3] There are numerous safety issues here, and this treatment should only be undergone under the supervision of a qualified healthcare practitioner. Guidance from a healthcare practitioner is necessary to assure safety, determine proper dosage, prevent serious side effects or drug/supplement interactions, and to determine whether the patient is a suitable candidate for this treatment at all. Legal issues with psilocybin must also be considered, and they vary based on jurisdiction.

Please refer to the section on lithium for more information. In this author's personal experience and opinion, low-dosage lithium may be beneficial in OCD treatment. Again, a qualified healthcare practitioner must guide treatment to assure safety, prevent drug/supplement interactions, determine proper dosage, and to ascertain the suitability of the patient for treatment with lithium.

Neurofeedback may have potential in the treatment of OCD. In my personal experience, however, it was not a "cure" for the condition. In the big picture, I was a bit disappointed with neurofeedback's efficacy for me, but everyone's outcome is different. Some people seem to have very positive experiences with neurofeedback, and it should not be dismissed in terms of being potentially beneficial in the neuropsychiatric space.

Inositol may have application in the treatment of OCD.[4] I have positive personal experience with inositol. Milk thistle (*Silybum marianum*) may have utility in obsessive-compulsive disorder.[5-7] Glycine and borage may also have utility in obsessive-compulsive disorder. NAC (N-Acetylcysteine) may also be considered as a potential option in OCD.[8] Again, a healthcare practitioner should be involved here to come up with a safe and individually tailored program for dealing with the OCD. Dosage, interactions, side effects, and patient suitability should be checked before proceeding. The utmost care must be taken to not create dangerous side effects through supplement interactions. Combining supplements/herbs which have similar mechanisms of action requires expertise to avoid potentially dangerous outcomes and should generally be avoided.

It is also recommended to do a deep psychotherapeutic exploration of childhood and potential trauma. Working through such issues, in addition to utilizing CBT, can help move toward healing of OCD. The work of Dr. Jeffrey M. Schwartz can be potentially very helpful in dealing with OCD. The type of cognitive changes recommended by Dr. Schwartz seem necessary toward healing OCD. But for people with internal compulsions, sometimes they need to get the situation under control to make it easier to actually do this cognitive work. The ideas presented in this section will hopefully provide support in helping the process of healing from OCD.

Parkinson's Disease

Eat a 100% whole-food organic plant-based diet with supplemental vitamin B12. Eliminate artificial colors, flavors, and preservatives. Eliminate trans fats. Eliminate added salt, oil, and sugar. Food intake should be derived as much as possible from raw, boiled, or steamed food while keeping high-temperature cooking (baking, frying) to a minimum. Avoiding high-temperature cooking minimizes exposure to acrylamide (a neurotoxin).

Ensure maximum sunshine exposure (but avoid sunburn). Avoid shift work. Consider water-only fasting, which may be helpful (see "Fasting" section above for precautions/contraindications). Results from fasting in this particular condition may be disappointing. However, fasting still has profoundly beneficial effects on overall health. Ensure adequate and appropriate physical activity based on the individual health situation. Eat 100% organic and live an organic and ecological lifestyle to minimize exposure to toxins (including neurotoxins). Avoid lead (old paint, water piping, etc.) and mercury (dental amalgam, fish, coal-burning power plants, broken fluorescent light bulbs, old thermometers, etc.).

Minimize exposure to electromagnetic fields. Avoid cellphone use. Avoid wireless telephones. Utilize corded landlines and wired internet cables and routers. If cellphone use is necessary keep it at a maximum distance from the body and use the phone's speaker. Keep general technology use to a minimum. Minimize technology in the bedroom and keep electromagnetic field exposure as low as possible.

Addressing issues related to Mind-Body Medicine including stress management, positive thinking, increasing social support, healing past trauma, prayer, and spirituality may be beneficial.

The following plants may have utility in Parkinson's Disease: *Allium sativum, Bacopa monnieri, Brassica oleracea, Camelia sinensis, Centella asiatica, Chamaemelum nobile* or *Matricaria chamomilla, Cinnamomum verum, Cuminum cyminum, Curcuma longa, Hericium erinaceus, Hypericum perforatum, Nigella sativa, Passiflora spp., Phyllanthus emblica, Punica granatum, Rosmarinus officinalis, Scutellaria baicalensis, Scutellaria lateriflora, Syzygium aromaticum, Vaccinium myrtillus, Zingiber officinale.*

Please refer to the individual herb listings and other mentioned sections of this work for details, references, and important precautions.

Post-Traumatic Stress Disorder (Trauma Healing including for Post-Traumatic Stress Disorder (PTSD) and Complex PTSD)

Trauma Healing is fundamental to achieving overall health and wellness. There are numerous options for addressing trauma. It is beyond the scope of this work to go into details about every option. However, a broad look at some of the options can give hope and an introduction to what is available to help on the path of healing. Every person is unique. There is not one correct path for everyone. However, the presentation of all of these various options and ideas will likely accelerate people's ability to find the right path for them.

Dr. James S. Gordon's work offers numerous ideas for healing from trauma.[1] What is particularly appealing about Dr. Gordon's work is that he presents minimal-cost treatments as options. The low cost makes these options widely available, and they can be implemented on a broad scale when dealing with large-scale traumas that affect many people simultaneously. Dr. Gordon's book is highly recommended, as well as the associated website[2] for the Center for Mind-Body Medicine, which provides videos and resources to help implement these healing strategies. Treatment options include Meditation (called Soft Belly by Dr. Gordon), Drawings (creating hope through Art), Shaking and then Dancing, Emotional Expression (through the use of a Journal or having a dialogue with your emotion(s)), social support (including individual therapy, group therapy, support groups, friends or family), using imagery to connect with your inner wisdom, taking baths, massage, exercise, punching pillows, spending time in nature, spending time with animals, laughter, learning about your family history, practicing gratitude, forgiveness, love, and finding purpose and meaning in life. EMDR (Eye Movement Desensitization and Reprocessing), Somatic Experiencing, and Dialectical Behavior Therapy (DBT) are among the other therapies discussed by Dr. Gordon to treat trauma.

As Dr. Gordon discusses gratitude, the idea comes up that gratitude leads to happiness. This idea is so simple yet profound. Practicing gratitude can dramatically increase happiness. This is a vital lesson and should be incorporated into daily life. I personally find that knowing this information in theory is not sufficient to increase happiness. Accessing, actually experiencing, the *feeling* of gratitude, is extremely important. The feeling of it, the energy of that feeling, can completely change the way someone sees their life. Feeling grateful leads to happiness. And I believe virtually anyone, under wonderful conditions and also under the most difficult circumstances imaginable, can focus on one tiny thing to feel gratitude about in that moment. It really can transform life in a more positive direction. Gratitude, meaning in life, purpose, authenticity, self-love, love in general, social connection, and serving a purpose greater than just caring for yourself-these are profoundly important concepts that move us toward happiness and inner peace.

The Shaking/Dancing exercise is really simple and is wonderful for the nervous system of people with unresolved trauma. Animals release trauma through shaking, and humans are animals. I find this method quite useful. This exercise allows us to directly access our instinct for processing trauma. For more information on shaking and how animals heal from trauma, consult the work of Dr. Peter Levine, the creator of Somatic Experiencing. In general, the idea of Somatic Experiencing is that trauma is stored in the body, and through accessing and focusing on sensations in the body, one can hopefully process and release the trauma. There is a high value placed on sensations and feelings.

EMDR (Eye Movement Desensitization and Reprocessing) is a highly effective method of treating trauma. Francine Shapiro created this method of treatment that can be profoundly useful in trauma therapy. The treatment can be done in various ways, including tapping, following the therapist's finger movement, etc. The eye movement from side to side (with other variations possible) and the shift in sensory focus from side to side while focusing on particular thoughts/memories seem to facilitate healing. This form of healing may possibly be related to the

Rapid Eye Movement (REM) in sleep/ dreaming. In any case, the life work of the late Dr. Francine Shapiro has been instrumental to trauma therapy.

Dr. Bessel Van Der Kolk, in the powerful book *The Body Keeps the Score*, discusses therapeutic options for treating trauma, including Yoga, theater (acting and expression), neurofeedback, EMDR (Eye Movement Desensitization and Reprocessing), hypnosis, MDMA, massage, LSD, acupuncture, writing, musical therapy, art therapy, dance therapy, psychomotor therapy, and internal family systems therapy.[3]

I want to add some personal thoughts regarding neurofeedback. This therapy involves doing a quantitative EEG to detect abnormal brain wave patterns in various regions of the brain and then utilizing mental training in an attempt to correct those wave patterns. After a series of treatments is concluded, a post-series quantitative EEG is repeated to see if the brain-wave patterns have shifted. My personal experience with neurofeedback was disappointing in terms of overall results. However, I do believe that neurofeedback may be beneficial in certain patients. I have come to believe that neurofeedback may be a bit of a superficial treatment in some ways —an underlying issue certainly created the abnormal brain waves, and training that corrects the brain wave patterns may not heal the underlying cause. In that sense, it may be a cosmetic fix. However, correcting the brain wave patterns may also be enough of a stimulus to actually foster profound growth in terms of healing from other pathways (therapy, etc.). It is not my intent to discourage this therapy, but only to mention possible limitations on success. I do not think it is enough alone to heal trauma without other inner work being done.

I do believe yoga has great use in treating trauma and should be incorporated into someone's routine if at all possible. Hypnosis also can be useful in facilitating the healing of trauma. Caution is advised with hypnosis, in particular with choosing a therapist. The therapist really needs to be skilled and have deep empathy and sensitivity. In my opinion, a skilled hypnotherapist can facilitate trauma healing. However, the absence of sufficient skill in hypnosis, or the lack of empathy and sensitivity to the client, may potentially worsen symptoms. There is risk here, and also potential rewards with the right hypnotherapist.

Psychedelic therapy clearly has a place in trauma treatment but must be done under proper supervision (with available psychological guidance and medical backup if necessary). The legal framework for such therapy is constantly changing and is clearly an issue that must be carefully considered on a case-by-case basis. There is great potential in this avenue of treatment, but I believe it is important not to believe that one can only heal by using an external substance. There are multiple ways to heal, and healing is possible without external substances. These substances can, however, facilitate access to something hidden inside us. That being the case, the obvious utility of psychedelic therapy in trauma treatment requires that it be considered as a valuable option in this field.

Pete Walker's work is also beneficial in navigating the path of healing from trauma.[4] He offers numerous tools and concepts that can guide people toward healing Complex PTSD.

Incorporating Gabor and Daniel Maté's work will maximize the chances of healing.[5] Addressing issues such as authenticity, compassion, healthy anger, boundaries, and disease as a message from the body are vital components of healing. In addition, the work discusses the therapeutic potential of psychedelic treatments in terms of trauma/addiction.

Utilizing meditations from Dr. Joe Dispenza can be profoundly beneficial.[6-7] In fact, these meditations can open something that may lead to incredible shifts in life and healing. The disconnection and dissociation that may come with trauma separates us from ourselves and those around us. Reconnecting with love, which can happen through Dr. Dispenza's meditation exercises, may be the beginning of healing. To feel love is important and healing.

Mónica de Sá is a gifted psychologist and trauma therapist who practices in Barcelos and Porto, Portugal.[8] She shared the important wisdom with me that the core of trauma healing involves self-love and self-acceptance.[9] If this is really the core of trauma healing, then using Dr. Joe Dispenza's meditation to feel love, while simultaneously visualizing yourself as a child and directing love toward that child, can be an important step. Imagine that child version of yourself being loved deeply and growing into your current adult self and keep feeling that love toward yourself. It is important to really focus on self-love and self-acceptance, and then branch out into love of others. Of course, feeling unity and connection with the world and universe around us is also healing, and finding meaning and purpose in life (and serving something greater than yourself) is of the utmost value. I feel it is important to add that for people really disconnected from their feelings and their bodies, it can be difficult to feel love in general. Sometimes it is easier to start by feeling love for someone else, and then later on focusing love on yourself. If self-love is really missing, it can be particularly beneficial to start the process by feeling love for your child (if you have a child) or for an animal companion. This incredible love can easily be adapted to help achieve self-love later on. The concepts of unity and connection make it important to simply start the process of connecting with love and then expanding that concept to yourself and others.

Another important tool shared by trauma therapist Monica de Sá involves imagining inserting your own story into someone else's life (your child or someone you deeply love would be especially useful).[9] In many cases, you may feel tremendous empathy for the other person in this mental exercise. And yet, the same story in you brings about shame, guilt, and a lack of compassion/love/acceptance. The idea, of course, is to treat yourself with the same love, compassion, and acceptance that you would the other person. All of this work helps create self-love and self-acceptance, which creates a strong foundation for healing.

I believe that using water in the treatment of trauma can accelerate the healing process. It seems to have the ability to reduce dissociation and bring one back into the body. Showers can be beneficial. Baths and swimming should also be considered. Of course, with all water work, there may be contraindications and precautions that prevent the safe application of water-based therapies. But when safely used, water can really make a profound difference in recovery from trauma. A unique and powerful option in facilitating trauma healing is Watsu.[10] This work involves a practitioner moving and holding the client in the water during the sessions. It can be incredibly relaxing and healing to the nervous system of someone with PTSD. Emotional release may occur during the sessions.

Another interesting water-based therapy is flotation in water with reduced sensory stimulation treatment (sometimes referred to as an isolation tank). While I do not have personal experience with this as of this writing, it is worth noting as possibly beneficial. Not only is water involved, but extremely high levels of magnesium are present in the treatment water, which may be uniquely beneficial in trauma treatment.[11]

In specific circumstances, additional vitamin or mineral supplementation beyond the general recommendations may be helpful. The general supplementation guidelines have been discussed elsewhere in this book, including vitamin B12 supplementation. Ensuring adequate vitamin B12 intake is necessary for everyone. Here, the aim is to discuss some other nutritional issues related to neurological and psychological health. Some people with neuropsychological symptoms, including PTSD, may benefit from supplementation with vitamin B6 and zinc.[12] In specific circumstances, niacin supplementation may be beneficial for both neurological and psychological health, but there are safety considerations, and each case must be dealt with on an individual basis.[13] Magnesium may be beneficial in supporting people with PTSD.

Lithium is a profoundly important mineral in terms of neurological and psychological health. It is likely an essential mineral, and a recommended intake of 1 mg per 70 kg of body weight has been suggested.[14] At a minimum, a deficiency in the mineral should be avoided. The effects on the brain are so profound that this issue needs further elaboration. The brain-protecting benefits of lithium may be beneficial in a wide variety of psychological and neurological issues.[15-17] Depression, anxiety, violence, rage, post-traumatic stress disorder, Alzheimer's, Parkinson's, and addiction are some of the issues in which lithium may have a positive effect. Many of the side effects and the bad reputation of lithium are associated with the higher dosages used in conventional psychiatry. When carefully used in the right patients in the lowest effective dosage, side effects can generally be minimized or in many cases eliminated completely. It is best to work with a qualified healthcare practitioner to avoid drug interactions and to determine if lithium is safe for you. Lithium may be contraindicated in some medical conditions. In addition, people with kidney and thyroid conditions must always exercise caution with respect to lithium usage. And some people are simply sensitive to lithium, even at relatively low dosages. But in carefully selected people who are monitored by a qualified healthcare practitioner, low-dosage lithium may be extremely beneficial in a wide variety of mental and neurological health conditions. Depending on weight and the specific individual's health condition, the dosage of elemental lithium may vary in adults from a few hundred micrograms per day to 1 mg per day, to 5 mg, to 10 mg, to 40 mg per day. In general, up to 40 mg per day is safe, but not for everyone. Again, a person's sensitivity, any potential drug and supplement interactions, and underlying health conditions must be checked to ensure safety when using lithium, even at lower dosages. I want to emphasize the profound potential utility of using lithium, in appropriate patients, when treating PTSD. It has the potential to address PTSD through multiple mechanisms of action.

In general, the addition of supplementation should be done carefully and after consultation with a qualified healthcare practitioner who can assure safety in terms of dosage and prevent any harmful interactions with drugs or other supplements. This statement is not meant to necessarily discourage use, but rather to maximize safety, as each individual has their own health history, medication use, etc., which should be taken into consideration before utilizing these supplements.

An additional potentially beneficial option in dealing with trauma involves the work of Wim Hof.[18] The breathing exercises and cold exposure may have potential in terms of healing the nervous system from trauma. Specifically, the autonomic nervous system may be positively impacted, and this would be an important benefit for people dealing with unresolved trauma. There are contraindications and precautions related to the Wim Hof system, so please check with a qualified healthcare provider to ensure safety before deciding to proceed. It should be emphasized that one should never do the breathing exercises while in water, because drowning and death are possible. Do not do the breathing exercises while driving or in the shower. This method has risks, and I hesitated to include it in this work. If you decide to incorporate it into your routine, do it at your own risk, only with maximum precautions and having checked with your healthcare provider first. All that being said, I personally feel it has been beneficial for me.

I want to add that trauma, PTSD, complex PTSD, and stress can serve as a starting point for chronic disease. The negative effects of chronic stress are well known and can lead to serious disease. Unresolved trauma negatively impacts the nervous system. It has been observed by Dr. Dietrich Klinghardt that more trauma tends to correlate with more toxins in the body. Stress also negatively impacts the immune system. An imbalance in the parasympathetic/ sympathetic nervous system due to trauma can have a profoundly negative impact on health. Healing will be impaired. Thus, whether through increased toxin accumulation, lack of detoxification, sleep deprivation, immune system impact, or other possible mechanisms, unresolved trauma can set the stage for serious chronic diseases. Of course, do not stress about this. Just plan to calmly address any unresolved trauma. I also want to strongly recommend that in the case of developmental trauma and complex PTSD, one seeks the guidance of a therapist trained in the NeuroAffective Relational Model™. This model has a comprehensive approach toward developmental trauma and complex PTSD.[19-20]

In conclusion, the treatment of trauma must receive the high priority that it deserves.

Schizophrenia

Eat a 100% whole-food organic plant-based diet with supplemental vitamin B12. Eliminate artificial colors, flavors, and preservatives. Eliminate trans fats. Eliminate added salt, oil, and sugar. Food intake should be derived as much as possible from raw, boiled, or steamed food while keeping high-temperature cooking (baking, frying) to a minimum. Avoiding high-temperature cooking minimizes exposure to acrylamide (a neurotoxin).

Ensure optimal sunshine exposure (but avoid sunburn). Avoid shift work. Consider water-only fasting, which may be profoundly useful (see specific section above for precautions/contraindications). In fact, fasting should be considered one of the most effective therapies for schizophrenia. Ensure adequate and appropriate physical activity based on the individual health situation. Eat 100% organic and live an organic and ecological lifestyle to minimize exposure to toxins (including neurotoxins). Avoid lead (old paint, water piping, etc.) and mercury (dental amalgam, fish, coal-burning power plants, broken fluorescent light bulbs, old thermometers, etc.).

Minimize exposure to electromagnetic fields. Avoid cellphone use. Avoid wireless telephones. Utilize corded landlines and wired internet cables and routers. If cellphone use is necessary, keep it at a maximum distance from the body and use the phone's speaker. Keep general technology use to a minimum. Minimize technology in the bedroom and keep electromagnetic field exposure as low as possible.

Addressing issues related to Mind-Body Medicine including stress management, positive thinking, increasing social support, healing past trauma, prayer, and spirituality may be beneficial.

I want to emphasize the importance of exploring the issue of unresolved trauma in schizophrenia. The writing of Dr. Abram Hoffer, and Orthomolecular Medicine in general, may be useful. See also the section on trauma ("Post-Traumatic Stress Disorder") above.

The following plants may have utility in schizophrenia: *Allium sativum, Bacopa monnieri, Brassica oleracea, Camelia sinensis, Centella asiatica, Chamaemelum nobile* or *Matricaria chamomilla, Cinnamomum verum, Curcuma longa, Ginkgo biloba, Hypericum perforatum, Nigella sativa, Phyllanthus emblica, Punica granatum, Scutellaria baicalensis, Scutellaria lateriflora, Syzygium aromaticum, Vaccinium myrtillus, Zingiber officinale.*

Please refer to the individual herb listings and other mentioned sections of this work for details, references, and important precautions.

Stroke

Eat a 100% whole-food organic plant-based diet with supplemental vitamin B12. Eliminate artificial colors, flavors, and preservatives. Eliminate trans fats. Eliminate added salt, oil, and sugar. Food intake should be derived as much as possible from raw, boiled, or steamed food while keeping high-temperature cooking (baking, frying) to a minimum. Avoiding high-temperature cooking minimizes exposure to acrylamide (a neurotoxin).

Ensure optimal sunshine exposure (but avoid sunburn). Avoid shift work. Consider water-only fasting, which may be profoundly useful (see specific section above for precautions/contraindications). Ensure adequate and appropriate physical activity based on the individual health situation. Eat 100% organic and live an organic and ecological lifestyle to minimize exposure to toxins (including neurotoxins). Avoid lead (old paint, water piping, etc.) and mercury (dental amalgam, fish, coal-burning power plants, broken fluorescent light bulbs, old thermometers, etc.).

Minimize exposure to electromagnetic fields. Avoid cellphone use. Avoid wireless telephones. Utilize corded landlines and wired internet cables and routers. If cellphone use is necessary keep it at a maximum distance from the body and use the phone's speaker. Keep general technology use to a minimum. Minimize technology in the bedroom and keep electromagnetic field exposure as low as possible.

Addressing issues related to Mind-Body Medicine including stress management, positive thinking, increasing social support, healing past trauma, prayer, and spirituality may be beneficial.

The following plants may have utility in stroke: *Allium sativum, Bacopa monnieri, Brassica oleracea, Camelia sinensis, Centella asiatica, Chamaemelum nobile* or *Matricaria chamomilla, Cinnamomum verum, Curcuma longa, Ginkgo biloba, Hericium erinaceus, Hypericum perforatum, Nigella sativa, Phyllanthus emblica, Punica granatum, Rosmarinus officinalis, Scutellaria baicalensis, Vaccinium myrtillus, Zingiber officinale.*

Please refer to the individual herb listings and other mentioned sections of this work for details, references, and important precautions.

Traumatic Brain Injury

Eat a 100% whole-food organic plant-based diet with supplemental vitamin B12. Eliminate artificial colors, flavors, and preservatives. Eliminate trans fats. Eliminate added salt, oil, and sugar. Food intake should be derived as much as possible from raw, boiled, or steamed food while keeping high-temperature cooking (baking, frying) to a minimum. Avoiding high-temperature cooking minimizes exposure to acrylamide (a neurotoxin).

Ensure optimal sunshine exposure (but avoid sunburn). Avoid shift work. Consider water-only fasting, which may be profoundly useful (see specific section above for precautions/contraindications). Ensure adequate and appropriate physical activity based on the individual health situation. Eat 100% organic and live an organic and ecological lifestyle to minimize exposure to toxins (including neurotoxins). Avoid lead (old paint, water piping, etc.) and mercury (dental amalgam, fish, coal-burning power plants, broken fluorescent light bulbs, old thermometers, etc.).

Minimize exposure to electromagnetic fields. Avoid cellphone use. Avoid wireless telephones. Utilize corded landlines and wired internet cables and routers. If cellphone use is necessary, keep it at a maximum distance from the body and use the phone's speaker. Keep general technology use to a minimum. Minimize technology in the bedroom and keep electromagnetic field exposure as low as possible.

Addressing issues related to Mind-Body Medicine including stress management, positive thinking, increasing social support, healing past trauma, prayer, and spirituality may be beneficial.

The following plants may have utility in traumatic brain injury: *Allium sativum, Bacopa monnieri, Brassica oleracea, Camelia sinensis, Centella asiatica, Chamaemelum nobile* or *Matricaria chamomilla, Cinnamomum verum, Curcuma longa, Ginkgo biloba, Hericium erinaceus, Hypericum perforatum, Nigella sativa, Phyllanthus emblica, Punica granatum, Rosmarinus officinalis, Scutellaria baicalensis, Vaccinium myrtillus, Zingiber officinale.*

Please refer to the individual herb listings and other mentioned sections of this work for details, references, and important precautions.

CHAPTER 3 REFERENCES

Aerotoxic Syndrome:

1. Functional Neurology Institute. "Aerotoxic syndrome." Accessed August 2, 2023. https://www.fninstitute.com/en/complaints/brain-trauma/ aerotoxic-syndrome.

2. Aerotoxic Association. "Home." Published December 4, 2019. Accessed August 2, 2023. https://aerotoxic.org/.

3. FlightsFrom.com. "Worldwide routes and flights from all airports." Accessed August 2, 2023. https://www.flightsfrom.com/

4. Air Europa Fleet | Air Europa Portugal. Accessed August 2, 2023. https://www.aireuropa.com/pt/en/aea/aexperience/fleet.

5. Haines, G. "Does EasyJet's new filtration system suggest toxic cabin air really is an issue?" *The Telegraph.* https://www.telegraph.co.uk/travel/ news/does-easy-jets-new-filtration-system-suggest-toxic-cabin-air-really-is-an-issue/. Published September 18, 2017. Accessed August 2, 2023.

6. Srour, S. Customer Service EasyJet. April 3, 2022.

7. EasyJet. "Our fleet|easyJet." Published 2022. Accessed August 2, 2023. https://www.easyjet.com/en/help/boarding-and-flying/our-fleet.

8. Cambridge Mask Co. Accessed August 2, 2023. https://cambridgemask.com/.

9. Flight Aware. "Treatment – Stichting Fly Aware." Accessed August 2, 2023. https://flyaware.nl/en/treatment/.

Brain Fog, Dissociation, Functional Neurological Disorders, Psychogenic Illness:

1. Victoria State Government Better Health Channel. "Dissociation and dissociative disorders." www.betterhealth.vic.gov.au. Accessed August 1, 2023. https://www.betterhealth.vic.gov.au/health/conditionsandtreatments/dissociation-and-disso-ciative-disorders#what-is-dissociation.

2. Mayo Clinic. "Functional neurologic disorders/conversion disorder— Symptoms and causes." Published 2017. Accessed August 2, 2023. https://www.mayoclinic.org/diseases-conditions/conversion-disorder/ symptoms-causes/syc-20355197.

3. Sarno, JE. *The Divided Mind: The Epidemic of Mindbody Disorders.* Harper; 2006.

COVID-19-Related Neurological and Psychiatric Issues:

1. Kathrada, N, P Kory, T Lawrie, P Mccullough. "Spike Protein Detox Guide 2023." Accessed August 14, 2023. https://worldcouncilforhealth.org/wp-content/uploads/2023/03/SpikeProteinDetox_ENGLISH_V2FH.pdf.

Obsessive-Compulsive Disorder (OCD):

1. Shannahoff-Khalsa, D, RY Fernandes, CAB Pereira, et al. "Kundalini Yoga Meditation Versus the Relaxation Response Meditation for Treating Adults With Obsessive-Compulsive Disorder: A Randomized Clinical Trial." *Front Psychiatry.* 2019; 10: 793. Published 2019 Nov 11. Doi: 10.3389/ fpsyt.2019.00793.

2. Shannahoff-Khalsa, DS, LE Ray, S Levine, CC Gallen, BJ Schwartz, and JJ Sidorowich. "Randomized controlled trial of yogic meditation techniques for patients with obsessive-compulsive disorder." *CNS Spectr.* 1999; 4(12): 34-47. Doi: 10.1017/ s1092852900006805.

3. Ehrmann, K, JJB Allen, and FA Moreno. "Psilocybin for the Treatment of Obsessive-Compulsive Disorders." *Curr Top Behav Neurosci.* 2022; 56: 247-259. Doi: 10.1007/7854_2021_279.

4. Levine. J. "Controlled trials of inositol in psychiatry." *Eur Neuropsychopharmacol.* 1997; 7(2): 147-155. Doi: 10.1016/s0924-977x(97)00409-4.

5. Sarris, J, D Camfield, and M Berk. "Complementary medicine, self-help, and lifestyle interventions for obsessive-compulsive disorder (OCD) and the OCD spectrum: a systematic review." *J Affect Disord.* 2012; 138(3): 213-221. Doi: 10.1016/j.jad.2011.04.051.

6. Camfield, DA, J Sarris, M Berk. "Nutraceuticals in the treatment of obsessive-compulsive disorder (OCD): a review of mechanistic and clinical evidence." *Prog Neuropsychopharmacol Biol Psychiatry.* 2011; 35(4): 887-895. Doi: 10.1016/j.pnpbp.2011.02.011.

7. Sayyah, M, H Boostani, S Pakseresht, and A Malayeri. "Comparison of *Silybum marianum (L.) Gaertn.* with fluoxetine in the treatment of Obsessive-Compulsive Disorder." *Prog Neuropsychopharmacol Biol Psychiatry.* 2010; 34(2): 362-365. Doi: 10.1016/j.pnpbp.2009.12.016.

8. Li, F, MC Welling, JA, Johnson, et al. "N-Acetylcysteine for Pediatric Obsessive-Compulsive Disorder: A Small Pilot Study." *J Child Adolesc Psychopharmacol.* 2020; 30(1): 32-37. Doi: 10.1089/cap.2019.0041.

Trauma Healing:

1. Gordon, James S. *Transforming Trauma: Discovering Wholeness and Healing after Trauma.* London, Yellow Kite, 2021.

2. The Center for Mind-Body Medicine. "Resources Archive." *CMBM*, cmbm.org/self-care-resources/resource/. Accessed 17 July 2023.

3. van der Kolk, Bessel. *The Body Keeps the Score: Brain, Mind, and Body in the Healing of Trauma.* 2014. New York, Penguin Books, 2015.

4. Walker, Pete. *Complex PTSD: From Surviving to Thriving: A Guide and Map for Recovering from Childhood Trauma.* 2013. Azure Coyote, 2014.

5. Maté, Gabor, and Daniel Maté. *The Myth of Normal: Trauma, Illness, and Healing in a Toxic Culture.* London, Vermillion, 2022.

6. Dispenza, Joe. "GOLOV-20 Meditation (Official Video)." Www.youtube.com, 24 Apr. 2020, www.youtube.com/watch?v=FZXVix4TNOI. Accessed 17 July 2023.

7. —. "U•Inspire•Me Meditation (Official Video)." Www.youtube.com, 2 May 2020, www.youtube.com/watch?v=ax7GWg6KQbY. Accessed 17 July 2023.

8. de Sá, Mónica Alison. "Mónica de Sá | Psicologia Clínica | Psicoterapia." Accessed August 5, 2023. https://www.monicadesa.pt/.

9. —. Personal Communication.

10. WATSU® Aquatic Bodywork and Therapy. Accessed August 8, 2023. https://www.watsu.com/

11. Pall, Martin L. *Explaining "Unexplained Illnesses": Disease Paradigm for Chronic Fatigue Syndrome, Multiple Chemical Sensitivity, Fibromyalgia, Post-Traumatic Stress Disorder, Gulf War Syndrome, and Others.* 2007.

12. "Kryptopyrroluria (Pyrrole Disorder / Pyroluria)." *Epidemic Answers.* epidemicanswers.org/symptoms_and_diagnoses/kryptopyrroluriapyrrole-disorder-pyroluria/. Accessed 31 July 2023.

13. Saul, Andrew. "DoctorYourself.com: Andrew Saul's Natural Health Website." *www.doctoryourself.com.* Accessed 31 July 2023.

14. Schrauzer, GN. "Lithium: occurrence, dietary intakes, nutritional essentiality." *Journal of the American College of Nutrition.* 2002; 21(1): 14-21. Doi: https://doi.org/10.1080/07315724.2002.10719188.

15. Greenblatt, J, and K Grossmann. *Nutritional Lithium: A Cinderella Story: The Untold Tale of a Mineral That Transforms Lives and Heals the Brain.* CreateSpace Independent Publishing Platform; 2016.

16. Millar, M. *The Natural Mental Health Breakthrough.* 2017.

17. —. "Home. The Lithium Doctor." Published March 9, 2013. Accessed July 13, 2023. http://www.thelithiumdoctor.com/.

18. Hof, W. "Welcome to the Official Wim Hof Method Website." *Wimhofmethod.com.* Published 2019. Accessed September 14, 2023. https://www.wimhofmethod.com.

19. Lapierre A, and L Heller. Healing Developmental Trauma. Berkeley, CA: North Atlantic Books; 2012.

20. Home. NARM Training Institute. Accessed November 12, 2023. https://narmtraining.com/

CHAPTER 4

Public Policies

Public Policy Implications for Health

Law and policy at the local, state/provincial, regional, national, and international levels can make a significant difference throughout the world in terms of health. These policies can have a profound impact on people's health, including their neurological and psychological health. It is important to learn from positive examples throughout the world and to avoid repeating actions that have created negative health outcomes. Replicating legal and policy changes which improve health can lead to significant improvements in health for many people This chapter will discuss some of these health-supporting policies, in the hope that these positive examples can be enacted elsewhere. While much of this work has focused on individual treatments and choices, the legal and policy choices made by governments definitely impact individuals as well. Activists, political leaders, voters, and organizations can use this section to promote positive health impact policies on a larger scale. Referendums on specific issues related to health and environmental policies can also positively promote health and well-being.

Addiction and Criminal Justice

Criminal justice systems can increase people's suffering, their stress, and their health problems (including the negative neurological impact of stress) when they are cruel and lack compassion. Thoughtful criminal justice systems do the reverse.

Since addiction is clearly tied to trauma and stress (please see the work of Dr. Gabor Maté), the criminal justice system should be compassionate in dealing with addiction, for example. Fair criminal justice systems are never about revenge but instead are about justice, compassion, healing, reconciliation, rehabilitation, and of course, protecting the safety of the community. Activists and elected officials can affect public policy on this issue and effect profoundly positive changes for improving people's health and well-being (including neuropsychiatric health).

A wonderful example of moving toward a more beneficial criminal justice system in terms of addiction is the Constitution of Ecuador.[1] The constitution presents addiction as a public health issue and opposes criminalizing it. Portugal has also essentially ended the criminalization of addicts.[2] It should be noted that for maximum success, treating addiction as a public health issue should be combined with sufficient financial resources to support people's healing. Another country which provides a positive model on this issue is Uruguay. Again, it must be made clear, that while ending the criminalizing of addicts is a wonderful first step, it is not sufficient in and of itself. People require broad-based support in dealing with any past trauma and overcoming coexisting challenges. Trauma, poverty, stress, housing issues, and coexisting mental health conditions must be addressed. These require significant deployment of financial resources.

Climate Change

Why include climate change in a work about healing the brain? Well, the current climate crisis is connected to many health issues. Human beings evolved in particular climates, and the current extremes of temperature and weather conditions create stress. Neurological health is compromised by excessive stress. The climate crisis may impact crop production and lead to increasing starvation and nutritional deficiencies—and this will negatively impact neuropsychiatric health. Climate change can impact the availability of fresh water—and this can certainly negatively impact people's health. It is quite possible that catastrophic events will occur in the near future due to climate change. And this crisis may ultimately lead, in the most extreme outcome, to human extinction.[1] This is a real possibility. We certainly cannot have neurological health if we are extinct.

So what can be done? Project Drawdown is a fantastic resource for ideas on addressing climate change.[2] This resource allows individuals, corporations, governments, activists, public policy experts, politicians, and organizations to quickly see numerous detailed proposed solutions. While I may not agree with each solution (for example, the use of old-style traditional nuclear power seems unwise in the era of increasingly extreme weather events), the resource is vital overall for addressing the issue of climate change. One of the solutions, "Plant-rich diets," has been discussed throughout this work as being potentially beneficial for health-related reasons. It is encouraging to see this as a potential solution to climate change, as well.

The Beyond Oil & Gas Alliance is an important movement addressing climate change.[3] It is encouraging to see twelve governments (Washington State, Tuvalu, Wales, Vanuatu, Sweden, Ireland, Quebec, Portugal,

Greenland, Denmark, France, and Costa Rica) take such a positive stance regarding climate change. All governments worldwide should commit to maximum action on this issue.

The 4 per 1000 Initiative encourages the adoption of regenerative agriculture.[4] This is an important component of addressing climate change. Vietnam, the United Kingdom, Uruguay, Tunisia, Spain, Senegal, Norway, Portugal, Poland, New Zealand, Mexico, the Netherlands, Japan, Lebanon, Austria, Scotland, Argentina, Canada, Cambodia, Chile, Ireland, the Ivory Coast, Hungary, Denmark, Germany, Estonia, France, and Finland are among the governments which have joined. Again, all governments worldwide should join this initiative.

Electromagnetic Fields

Wireless radiation potentially has profound negative neurological and psychiatric effects.[1-2] Its possible impact on the blood-brain barrier is seriously concerning. In fact, artificial electromagnetic fields are highly problematic in terms of overall health.[3-5] For more information about this issue, consult the Environmental Health Trust.[6]

On an individual level, one can minimize all use of wireless technology and replace it with wired options whenever possible. Using a wired home phone instead of a cell phone whenever possible is beneficial. Wired internet should be preferred over wireless. Avoid Bluetooth, cellphones, wireless routers, etc. Switch phones to airplane mode and deactivate wi-fi, mobile data, etc., whenever possible. Children should be protected as much as possible from this radiation.

In addition, avoiding fluorescent lighting is encouraged. Incandescent light bulbs appear to be the healthiest form of artificial lighting, despite using more electricity. Having a 100% renewable electric grid and healthy lighting is the ideal combination. Healthy lighting maximizes the use of natural light and when necessary, supplements with the healthiest artificial light available. The issue of blue light is also of concern. Installation of software which addresses blue light may help with this issue, for example Iris software.[7]

Switzerland, Italy, and Russia are examples of countries with strong protective regulations regarding wireless radiation.[8] Numerous countries have taken various actions on the issue of wireless radiation. For example, Israel, France, and Cyprus have addressed the issue of wireless technology in elementary schools. Activists, public policy, and elected officials can make a big difference on this issue. Regulations matter, and they can impact large populations. Maximizing neurological and psychiatric health depends on this issue being addressed properly.

Fluoride

Fluoride is potentially neuro-toxic and is not an essential nutrient.[1-2] This substance should not be added to water or salt. I recommend avoiding fluoridated toothpaste, fluoride supplements, fluoridated salt, and fluoridated water. One can have excellent dental health without adding fluoride. Public policy should not favor adding fluoride to the water or salt supply. Worldwide, 25 countries have some type of water fluoridation program. All other countries do not. In fact, 95% of humans worldwide drink non-fluoridated water. Salt fluoridation is very common in Germany and Switzerland.[3] In total, approximately 50 countries worldwide practice salt fluoridation.[4] Any effort at legislation, referendums, or public policy which eliminate water and salt fluoridation should be supported.

Food Irradiation

Food irradiation is touted by proponents as increasing food safety, reducing infestation, and reducing food-borne illness.[1] It is currently permitted in some form in at least 60 countries. However, the long-term safety of this process cannot be proven, and it certainly does not seem to be compatible with processes that have a long historical usage in terms of the human evolutionary time frame. The precautionary principle is warranted here and also an attempt to respect nature as much as possible. A world that seeks to maximize health in general and neurological health in particular would not risk the unknown potential long-term effects of ingesting irradiated food.

The practice of food irradiation does appear to be restricted in Austria, Sweden, and Luxembourg.[2-4] In addition, the practice also appears to be restricted in countries such as Bolivia, Columbia, Guyana, Suriname, Mongolia, Kazakhstan, Morocco, Libya, Mali, Chad, the Democratic Republic of Congo, Angola, and Namibia.[4-5] While regulations constantly change, at the time of this writing, these are examples to model in moving forward on this issue on the worldwide level. Public policy, elections, referendums, and activists can make a difference by moving toward the elimination of the practice of food irradiation. Food safety, preservation methods, and microbial contamination control should use more traditional methods that have a long history of safety.

Genetically Modified Organisms (GMOs)

Genetically modified organisms in the food supply and environment have been a controversial issue. Again, this is a technology which does not correspond with our natural evolutionary history as humans. The long-term potential risks are enormous. The precautionary principle must come into play for both overall and neurological health. On an individual level, it is recommended to avoid genetically modified organisms (GMOs) by consuming organic foods. Labeling for non-GMO products also helps guide dietary choices on the individual level.

Venezuela, Ecuador, and Peru have stringent restrictions on GMOs.[1] In fact, Ecuador's constitution makes clear that it favors the country being free from GMOs. Zimbabwe, Zambia, and Tanzania have more protective positions in terms of regulation of GMOs. New Zealand also has protective regulations regarding GMOs. In Europe, the law varies in each country.[2] Italy, for example, has a broad-based ban on GMO cultivation. These are positive examples to model elsewhere—in particular, the idea of including restrictions in the constitution (as in Ecuador). In fact, Ecuador's constitution includes respect for the rights of nature, a powerful concept. This concept can be utilized to legally protect people from various environmentally destructive activities (activities that otherwise could also damage human health).[3] Please refer to the Community Environmental Legal Defense Fund for further information on how respecting the rights of nature can be helpful in protecting people's health worldwide. The model can apply to GMO's, toxic chemicals, etc.

On the large-scale, big-picture level, collective action is very effective in terms of GMOs. Ideally, there would be a worldwide ban on any cultivation of genetically modified organisms for food. Public policy, elections, referendums, and activists should move toward eliminating GMOs from the food supply.

Glyphosate

Glyphosate is a chemical utilized as a crop desiccant and herbicide. It is potentially profoundly toxic and may have devastating effects on the human neurological system.[1] Minimizing the population's exposure to glyphosate is vital to maximizing neurological and psychological health, along with overall health.

Glyphosate has been banned in Bahrain, Fiji, Kuwait, Oman, Qatar, and Saudi Arabia.[2] There is strong momentum in France, Germany, Italy, Luxembourg, and Mexico toward ending glyphosate use.

This chemical should be banned worldwide, and activists and policymakers should work toward this goal. Elections and referendums may help move us toward a global ban. People can work at the local, state/province, regional, national, and international levels on these issues. Since it is only one of many chemicals commonly used in agriculture, and the issue is much broader, replacing the entire system of agriculture with a more sustainable, organic, regenerative, permaculture-type system would solve the glyphosate issue, along with other issues.

Lead

Finland, Denmark, and Japan seem to have the lowest exposure to lead in the world.[1] Policies must be adopted to minimize and eliminate lead exposure. Lead should be eliminated wherever and whenever possible from the environment, including from paint, gasoline, piping, and lead solder. Lead contamination of food, whether through intentional adulteration or otherwise, needs to be aggressively addressed. PVC plastics, lead-based weapons, batteries, jewelry, ceramics, lipsticks, toys, and electronics are also products that need to be lead-free.[2] There should be a comprehensive analysis of lead levels and remediation of land with high levels. Lead is profoundly toxic, and comprehensively addressing this issue is vital to neurological and overall health.

Mercury Amalgam Fillings

Mercury is extremely neurotoxic and should be avoided whenever possible. The presence of mercury in mercury amalgam dental fillings is of serious concern. Any policy, legislation, or public movement away from mercury amalgam fillings should be supported. Positive examples include ending the use of amalgam in the Philippines, Moldova, Saint Kitts and Nevis, Norway, Sweden, and New Caledonia.[1-2] On the individual level, please refer to the International Academy of Oral Medicine and Toxicology for information regarding the safe removal of mercury amalgam fillings.[3]

Pesticide Use

As a general policy toward maximizing overall health, along with neurological health, organic, sustainable, regenerative, permaculture-style agriculture should be supported. Toxic pesticides should be banned. Sweden and France appear to have the most protective regulations in terms of pesticides.[1] These are positive models that protect people's health. The European Union in general and the UK also provide positive examples of pesticide protection. Brazil and Saudi Arabia also rank quite strongly in terms of pesticide regulations. And while bans and regulations are important, an overall move toward sustainable, regenerative, organic agriculture is also vital.

Poverty

Poverty may substantially increase a person's exposure to stress and have negative impacts on neuropsychiatric and overall health. Public policy, activism, and political leaders can focus on kindness and social support to help minimize poverty. Maximizing social support can be done in various ways. It is strongly preferred to create systems that are as supportive as possible while minimizing bureaucracy. That is, systems should be simple and easy to navigate. Bureaucracy and complexity increase people's stress. Creating numerous conditions for receiving support increases stress. So the goal should be to maximize support while minimizing stress and bureaucracy. This section does not claim to have all of the answers, but there are various possible options. Having a minimum wage which is a living wage, adjusted for inflation, may help reduce poverty.

Another option would be a universal, unconditional guaranteed income. It is really important that this income be unconditional. The danger, of course, is that authoritarian-minded people in power could abuse this system to coerce people into particular behaviors as a condition for receiving this income—this must not occur for the system to be ethical and just. If the universally guaranteed income came without any conditions, it could be an extremely helpful program to eliminate poverty. This guaranteed income should be available to all and without conditions. It should not be means-tested, which would only add to complexity and stress. The universal income idea would be a strong base for people to build on to pursue their own meaningful work. If the income were significant enough and the system design was unconditional and simple, it could replace a significant amount of the bureaucracy found in many governmental programs on every level. Society would have to decide that this program is a priority in order to fit it within a balanced budget. Increasing the money supply in order to pay for such programs would increase inflation, and inflation is highly problematic. The goal is to minimize poverty without increasing inflation. This requires shifting money from programs that are harmful to the universal income program. Another method for funding such a program without increasing the money supply would be to have a worldwide agreement between all nations that there is a maximum amount of wealth that each person can have—for example no more than 1 billion dollars of wealth total per person. Any assets above that amount could be redistributed to all people through the universal income program (even those extremely wealthy people would receive the universal income, obviously). This program would find more success if it operated on a worldwide basis. If it were only applied in one country, those billionaires would likely shift their wealth to a different country. People globally simply need to decide that there must be limits on individual wealth and power—and any wealth beyond the agreed limit must be redistributed equally to everyone (including to those wealthy individuals). Simplifying the output of that system (universal income) prevents bureaucracy. This type of universal income system may become even more desirable in the world of Artificial Intelligence and more and more advanced technology. Such a system could minimize poverty, crime, and stress and improve health, including neuropsychiatric health. It also would reduce the concentration of power and control and maximize democracy. Simultaneously, the chances for survival of the human species would improve on issues such as climate change (due to the improvement in democracy, reduced corruption, and reduced concentration of power/wealth/control).

Maslow's hierarchy of needs can be considered. Universal income is a wonderful start to making sure everyone's basic needs are met. Some of the more basic needs, such as housing, safety, food, water, financial resources, and healthcare (including physical and mental health) perhaps require government involvement. Charities, non-government organizations, religious organizations, and governments may need to work together to help people meet their basic needs. When everyone's basic needs are met, the entire society benefits. Stress levels should be reduced, in addition to crime being reduced. Neuropsychiatric health should benefit on the society-wide level.

Safe Public Drinking Water

Having clean and safe public drinking water available from the tap is vital to health. Having clean tap water that lacks residual disinfectant at the final point of consumption has potential health benefits. Countries that have moved toward the idea of not having residual disinfectant at the final point of consumption (when possible) include Austria, Germany, the Netherlands, and Switzerland.[1-4] This type of approach requires a big-picture approach to water quality throughout the entire system. Overall water quality, including minimizing and eliminating heavy metal exposure, pesticides, pharmaceutical drugs, and other toxins in water must be a priority. Providing high-quality water is a vital part of overall health, including neurological and psychological health. This issue must be a priority in elections, in public policy, and among activists.

Trans Fats

Partially hydrogenated oils are unnatural products that are destructive to overall health, including neurological health. Denmark was the first country in the world to protect their population from partially hydrogenated oils in 2004.[1] More recently, there has been a move toward a global ban on trans fats.[2] Significant progress has occurred on this issue in India, Bangladesh, Ukraine, the Philippines, Paraguay, Turkey, the European Union, the United Kingdom, Peru, Brazil, and Singapore. This is all good news, but it is important to mention that a massive number of deaths could have been prevented by acting earlier. Respecting nature and not creating this product in the first place would have been the best choice. And numerous deaths could have been avoided and significant health improvement could have occurred if Denmark's protective action had been modeled throughout the world in 2004. This is something to keep in mind when considering harmful unnatural exposures in our modern world and their impact on health. Activism and public policy matter deeply.

Vaccination

The issue of vaccination cannot be avoided in a discussion on neurological health. This issue is extremely complicated, and it is beyond the scope of this work to go into detail on this topic. There are issues of vaccine safety testing, ingredients, side effects, efficacy, individual versus community benefits/side effects, issues of bodily autonomy and freedom of choice, mandatory vaccinations versus optional, the risks of infectious diseases, overall benefits versus benefits in preventing the specific disease, and overall harm versus potential benefit in reducing the target disease, etc.

This issue has become extremely politicized, which is unfortunate. Regardless of whether an idea is true or false, a person belonging to one political group may go along with it because it is part of their party's stance, regardless of what they actually would believe if they studied the issue in depth.

I do not want to make any recommendations regarding what people should do in terms of vaccinating themselves or their children. This issue is complex and everyone needs to decide for themselves what is best. Infectious diseases can be deadly, and certainly, these diseases can have negative neuropsychiatric effects. On the other hand, there are serious potential safety concerns related to vaccination in terms of adverse neurological consequences. Unfortunately, this issue has become so controversial that saying anything that questions the conventional wisdom can have serious consequences for someone's livelihood and reputation. And while I will not make recommendations about what people should do in terms of vaccination on the individual level, I do think something so intimately tied to health (including neurological health) needs to be discussed.

The freedom to decide what to put into our bodies is sacred. No government should ever be allowed to force or pressure us to comply with a medical procedure. It is clear that this human right of bodily freedom was violated during the COVID-19 pandemic. It is also being violated with vaccination mandates for school entry throughout the world.[1] Regardless of the debate around vaccine safety and efficacy, mandatory vaccination violates human rights. Vaccination is not mandatory for school entry in many places throughout the world, such as Bolivia, Portugal, Spain, Ireland, the United Kingdom, Iceland, Denmark, the Netherlands, Norway, Sweden, Finland, Russia, India, and Kenya. This data is from 2019, so it should be interpreted with caution due to the effect of COVID-19 on vaccination policies. COVID-19 vaccination policies violated human rights in many parts of the world.[2]

Vaccine safety also needs to improve. Vaccine ingredients should be examined and cleaned up as much as possible. The entire vaccination process should replicate a natural infection as much as possible but with lower risk, obviously. Please refer to Children's Health Defense for important details regarding the vaccination issue.[3] It would be excellent to have safe vaccines that minimize the risk of side effects and provide high efficacy against dangerous infectious diseases. To help us get there, we need to have an honest discussion about this issue. Things can't improve without admitting that there may be a problem.

Again, I am not telling anyone what to do regarding vaccines. Infectious diseases can be deadly, and you assume that risk if you decide to avoid vaccination. Maintaining optimal nutritional status, good sanitation, and avoiding overcrowding can reduce risk. But there are risks to avoiding vaccination even in the best of circumstances. Those risks need to be compared to the risk of the vaccine itself. Homeopathic vaccination is an option worth looking into. It was used successfully in Cuba against leptospirosis, for example.[4] People can utilize various options in naturopathic medicine to support themselves during infectious diseases. But, depending on the specific disease, there can be a huge risk to avoiding the vaccination. It is an individual's responsibility to investigate this issue and decide the correct course of action for themself. The consequences of the decision in terms of the individual's health must be accepted by the individual. In conclusion, this issue is very complex. People should demand maximum safety in terms of vaccinations. They should have the freedom to decide for themselves what to do. And they should accept the consequences of their decision on their individual health (including neurological health), regardless of whether they decide to vaccinate or not.

CHAPTER 4 REFERENCES

Addiction and Criminal Justice:

1. Constitute Project. "Ecuador 2008 (rev. 2021) Constitution." Accessed August 17, 2023. https://www.constituteproject.org/constitution/Ecuador_2021?lang=en.

2. Inspire Malibu. "10 Countries That Ended Their War on Drugs" Published January 8, 2018. Accessed August 17, 2023. https://www.inspiremalibu.com/blog/drug-addiction/10-countries-that-ended-their-war-on-drugs/.

Climate Change:

1. Bendell, Jem. "Prof Jem Bendell." Published August 15, 2023. Accessed August 18, 2023. https://jembendell.com/.

2. Project Drawdown. "Table of Solutions." Published February 5, 2020. Accessed August 18, 2023. https://www.drawdown.org/solutions/table-of-solutions.

3. Beyond Oil & Gas Alliance. Accessed August 18, 2023. https://beyondoilandgasalliance.org/.

4. 4 per 1000. "Home." Accessed August 18, 2023. https://4p1000.org/?lang=en.

Electromagnetic Fields:

1. Bioinitiative.org. "Reported Biological Effects from Radiofrequency Radiation at Low-Intensity Exposure (Cell Tower, Wi-Fi, Wireless Laptop and "Smart" Meter RF Intensities)." Accessed August 18, 2023. https://bioinitiative.org/wp-content/uploads/pdfs/BioInitiativeReport-RF-Color-Charts.pdf.

2. Environmental Health Trust. "Scientific Research on Wireless Radiation Health Effects." Accessed August 18, 2023. https://ehtrust.org/science/wireless-radiation-health-effects/.

3. Mercola, J. *EMF*D: 5G, Wi-Fi & Cell Phones: Hidden Harms and How to Protect Yourself.* Hay House; 2020.

4. Rees, C, and M Havas. *Public Health SOS.* CreateSpace Independent Publishing Platform; 2009.

5. Davis, D. *Disconnect.* Dutton; 2010.

6. Environmental Health Trust. "Education, Research, and Policy to Reduce Environmental Risks." Accessed August 18, 2023. https://ehtrust.org/.

7. Georgiev, D. "Protect your Eyes. Be Healthy. Achieve more | Iris." *iristech.co.* Accessed August 18, 2023. https://iristech.co/.

8. Environmental Health Trust. "Database of Worldwide Policies on Cell Phones, Wireless and Health." Accessed August 18, 2023. https://ehtrust.org/policy/international-policy-actions-on-wireless/.

Fluoride:

1. Connett, PH, JS Beck, and HS Micklem. *The Case Against Fluoride: How Hazardous Waste Ended up in Our Drinking Water and the Bad Science and Powerful Politics That Keep It There.* Chelsea Green Pub; 2010.

2. Fluoride Action Network. "F.A.Q." Published December 15, 2011. Accessed August 14, 2023. https://fluoridealert.org/faq/.

3. Götzfried, F. "Legal aspects of fluoride in salt, particularly within the EU." *ForschungWissenschaft.* 2006; 116: 371-375. Accessed August 14, 2023. https://www.fluoridealert.org/wp-content/uploads/gotzfried-2006.pdf.

4. Alliance for a Cavity-Free Future. "Salt Fluoridation." Accessed August 14, 2023. https://www.acffglobal.org/salt-fluoridation/.

Food Irradiation:

1. International Atomic Energy Assn. "Food irradiation, benefits, use, standards | IAEA." *Iaea.org.* Published April 13, 2016. Accessed August 14, 2023. https://www.iaea.org/topics/food-irradiation.

2. Ehlermann, D. "Regulations Related to Trading of Irradiated Food in European Countries." *Iaea.org.* Accessed August 14, 2023. https://inis.iaea.org/ collection/ NCLCollectionStore/_Public/30/031/30031641.pdf?r=1&r=1.

3. Eur.lex. "List of Member States' authorisations of food and food ingredients which may be treated with ionising radiation (According to Article 4(6) of Directive 1999/2/EC of the European Parliament and of the Council on the approximation of the laws of the Member States concerning foods and food ingredients treated with ionising radiation)" Published 2009. Accessed August 15, 2023. https://eur-lex.europa.eu/legal-content/EN/ ALL/?uri=CELEX:52009XC1124(02).

4. Center for Consumer Research. "Is This Technology Being Used in Other Countries?" Published June 28, 2017. Accessed August 14, 2023. https://ccr.ucdavis.edu/food-irradiation/technology-being-usedother-countries.

5. Saravana, SK. "Food Irradiation_S.K.Saravana." *www.slideshare.net*. Published June 8, 2012. Accessed August 14, 2023. https://www.slideshare.net/ saravanask/food-irradiationsksaravana#18.

Genetically Modified Organisms:

1. Turnbull, C, M Lillemo, and TAK Hvoslef-Eide. "Global Regulation of Genetically Modified Crops Amid the Gene Edited Crop Boom—A Review." *Frontiers in Plant Science.* 2021; 12. Doi: https://doi.org/10.3389/ fpls.2021.630396.

2. Gmo-free-regions.org. "Bans." Published 2009. Accessed August 15, 2023. https://www.gmo-free-regions.org/gmo-free-regions/bans.html.

3. CELDF. "Community Rights Pioneers Protecting Nature and Communities." *CELDF.* Accessed August 15, 2023. https://celdf.org/.

Glyphosate:

1. Bush, Z. "Glyphosate, Root Cause of Chronic Inflammation?" *zachbushmd.com*. Accessed August 15, 2023. https://zachbushmd.com/ wp-content/uploads/2017/04/Glyphosate-Article-for-Holistic-Primary-Care-3-21-16.pdf.

2. Wisner Baum. "Where is Glyphosate Banned?" Published May 2023. Accessed August 15, 2023. https://www.wisnerbaum.com/toxic-tort-law/ monsanto-roundup-lawsuit/where-is-glyphosate-banned-/.

Lead:

1. Environmental Performance Index. "Lead exposure." *epi.yale.edu*. Accessed September 8, 2023. https://epi.yale.edu/epi-results/2022/component/pbd.

2. Environment UN. "Lead: What are the sources of lead in the environment?" *UNEP - UN Environment Programme*. Published September 16, 2017. Accessed September 8, 2023. https://www.unep.org/resources/infographic/lead-what-are-sources-lead-environment.

Mercury Amalgam Fillings:

1. International Academy of Oral Medicine and Toxicology (IAOMT). "Position Paper against Dental Mercury Amalgam Fillings for Medical and Dental Practitioners, Dental Students, Dental Patients, and Policy Makers." Accessed August 14, 2023. https://iaomt.org/wp-content/uploads/ IAOMT-Position-Paper-on-Dental-Amalgam.pdf.

2. Mercola, J. "The Latest Updates on Mercury-Free Dentistry in Europe and around the World a Special Interview with Charlie Brown." Accessed August 14, 2023. https://mercola.fileburst.com/PDF/ExpertInterviewTranscripts/DrJosephMercola-CharlieBrown-TheLatestUpdatesOnMercuryFreeDentistryInEuropeAndAroundTheWorld.pdf.

3. The International Academy of Oral Medicine and Toxicology. *IAOMT.* Accessed August 15, 2023. https://iaomt.org/

Pesticide Use:

1. Pesticide Info. "Banned Pesticides." *www.pesticideinfo.org.* Accessed August 16, 2023. https://www.pesticideinfo.org/resources/banned-pesticides.

Public Water:

1. Winfield, S. "10 Countries With The Cleanest Water Ranked (Best and Worst)." *Water Defense.* Published July 13, 2022. Accessed August 14, 2023. https://water-defense.org/water/tap/countries-with-the-cleanest-water/.

2. Rosario-Ortiz F, J Rose, V Speight, U von Gunten, and J Schnoor. "How do you like your tap water?" *Science.* 2016; 351(6276): 912-914. Doi: 10.1126/ science.aaf0953.

3. Rosario-Ortiz, F, and V Speight. "Can drinking water be delivered without disinfectants like chlorine and still be safe?" *The Conversation.* Published March 7, 2016. Accessed August 14, 2023. https://theconversation.com/can-drinking-water-be-delivered-without-disinfectants-like-chlorine-and-still-be-safe-55476.

4. Fish, KE, N Reeves-McLaren, S Husband, and J Boxall. "Unchartered waters: the unintended impacts of residual chlorine on water quality and biofilms." *NPJ Biofilms and Microbiomes.* 2020; 6(1). Doi: https://doi.org/ 10.1038/s41522-020-00144-w.

Trans Fat:

1. Belluz, J. "The new global plan to eliminate the most harmful fat in food, explained." *Vox.* Published May 14, 2018. Accessed August 16, 2023. https://www.vox.com/science-and-health/2018/5/14/ 17346108/trans-fats-food-world-health-organization-bloomberg-gates.

2. UN News. "Countries with regulations against industrially produced trans fats tripled over the past year." Published December 7, 2021. Accessed August 16, 2023. https://news.un.org/en/story/2021/12/1107382.

Vaccination:

1. Our World in Data. "Which countries have mandatory childhood vaccination policies?" Published June 11, 2021. Accessed September 14, 2023. https://ourworldindata.org/childhood-vaccination-policies.

2. Buchholz, K. "Infographic: The Countries Where Vaccination Is Mandatory." *Statista Infographics.* Published February 8, 2022. Accessed September 14, 2023. https://www.statista.com/chart/25326/obligatory-vaccination-against-covid-19/.

3. Children's Health Defense. "Help Children's Health Defense and RFK, Jr. end the epidemic of poor health plaguing our children." *Children's Health Defense.* Published 2019. Accessed September 14, 2023. https://childrenshealthdefense.org/.

4. Bracho, G, E Varela, R Fernández, et al. "Large-scale application of highly-diluted bacteria for Leptospirosis epidemic control." *Homeopathy.* 2010; 99(3): 156-166. Doi: 10.1016/j.homp.2010.05.009.

CONCLUDING REMARKS

This work represents more than two decades of my own search for healing. I wanted to synthesize the most important ideas I've learned over the years about healing and gather them into one book. It is my deepest wish that you find this work healing for you and that it facilitates your journey toward wellness. I hope it reaches as many practitioners and patients as possible in order to maximize healing and minimize suffering. I hope that the application of the ideas within this work can dramatically accelerate healing in the world.

INDEX

ABOUT THE AUTHOR

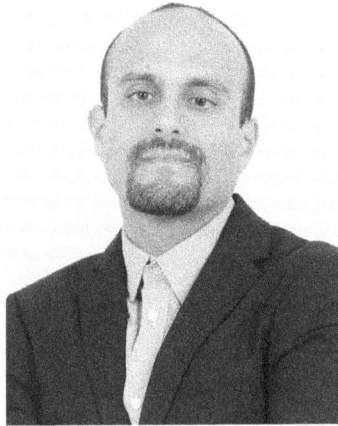

Shady J. Srour is a writer, herbalist, musician, activist, and father. His educational background is in Zoology (Animal Biology), Neuroscience, Herbal Medicine, and Plant-Based Nutrition. He enjoys hiking, yoga, and spending time with his children.

www.ingramcontent.com/pod-product-compliance
Lightning Source LLC
Chambersburg PA
CBHW041933260326
41914CB00010B/1278